GOOD MEDICINE

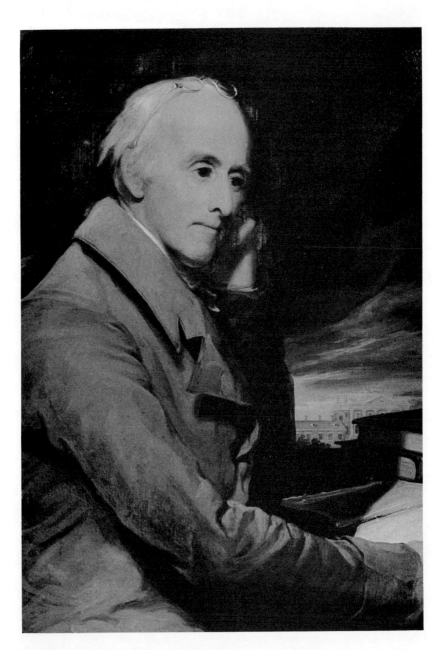

Benjamin Rush, M.D., 1746–1813.
(Portrait attributed to Thomas Sully)

GOOD MEDICINE

The First 150 Years of Rush-Presbyterian-St. Luke's Medical Center

Jim Bowman

CHICAGO REVIEW PRESS

All photos, unless otherwise credited, courtesy of Rush-Presbyterian-St. Luke's Medical Center.

ISBN: 1-55652-015-8 (cloth)
    1-55652-016-6 (paper)

LC No. 87-10305

Like the institution it chronicles, this book is dedicated "To the Glory of God and the Service of Man."

Contents

Prologue

This essay is meant not to close the book on Rush-Presbyterian-St. Luke's Medical Center but to open it. That is to say, it is an attempt at history by a writer who is not a historian in the hope that historians will have their interest piqued and others will find it a lively story.

If that sounds as if meant to disarm, let it. My approach has been to tell a story, though at times I have been more a mapper of landscape. In neither case have I tried to break new ground. Rather, I have leaned on others who did so—historians and other chroniclers, including journalists, who write history by the day.

It's a commemorative work in which I tried not to be too commemorative, lest readers feel called on more to praise famous men and women than to finish the book. I want readers to finish the book, though the table of contents and index will encourage browsing, which is all right too.

What I don't want is for readers to feel they have to read it because it describes a worthy cause (which it does). Hence it tells a story and moves as quickly as possible without footnotes and with a minimum of base-touching. The text itself has some footnote material.

At the end is a bibliography which expands what I say here, namely that I have written while standing on others' shoulders. There is also a list of interviewees. Maybe in the interview material a historian will find something to use. I am grateful to the interviewees, who helped me write the book.

I am also grateful to Bruce Rattenbury, who commissioned this book and shepherded it and me through the process of research, composition and approval. Pesky he wasn't, however, and for that I am doubly grateful. His associate Nancy K. Gallagher contributed editing help. William Kona, the Rush archivist, was very helpful in providing materials and verifying dates, titles and a dozen other details.

The advisory committee appointed by President Leo M. Henikoff, M.D., helped to flesh out my narrative. These are: Evan Barton, M.D., Doris Bolef M.L.S., Max Douglas Brown, J.D., Frederic de Peyster, M.D., Stanton A. Friedberg, M.D., the late Ruth Johnsen, R.N., Janet R. Kinney, M.D., C. Frederick Kittle, M.D., and again, William Kona. Erich E. Brueschke, M.D., provided helpful comment on the typescript, which was also read by Harold A. Kessler, M.D.

The usual disclaimer is in order: what's good is mine, what's bad is mine. Whatever you do, don't blame the advisors. In any event, I trust the book will tell you less than you want to know about a marvelously health-abetting enterprise preparing for its second 150 years.

Jim Bowman
February 1987

Rush is Chartered & Opened 1836–1857

The young surgeon Daniel Brainard came to Chicago in 1836 riding on a pony, one of many wise young men from the East who flooded into that village by the lake with streets of dust and mud and sidewalks made of wood. He was part of a human avalanche.

"Strangers fill our public houses and streets," said a local newspaper. "Our wharves are covered with men, women and children." Warehouses were thrown open to hold them. It was not unusual for 50 new immigrants to arrive in one day. One day, 200 came on 12 ships. Not a day passed with fewer than 10 arrivals. The village not yet a city numbered some 3,000 people.

Brainard himself was born in upstate New York, the fifth of nine children of a prosperous farmer. A tall, well built man, he was restless and ambitious.

He had studied at the small but influential College of Physicians and Surgeons at Fairfield, New York, as did Nathan S. Davis, later his colleague and competitor in Chicago. His Doctor of Medicine degree was from the highly respected Jefferson

1

Medical College in Philadelphia. As an Easterner, he was a typical newcomer to Chicago, where all but one of the first 10 mayors were Eastern-born.

Arriving in the village, he was met by John Dean Caton, a lawyer, whom he had known three years earlier when they were students in Rome, New York. On Caton's advice Brainard sold the pony to nearby Indians and deposited his saddle bags in Caton's office, there to begin his practice. It would do for a start.

He connected almost immediately with other physicians— movers and shakers of the community who shared his vision of a city served by well-educated doctors. The need was obvious. Sanitary, not to mention dietary, conditions were dismal. People didn't know how to eat or how to clean up after themselves. Thousands were crammed into tight spaces. A typical great American city was being born. Medicine was a high priority. Decent medical education was a must.

A medical school was in order, and no one knew it better than Brainard and these community leaders. In the fall of 1836, he and one of them, Dr. Josiah Goodhue, the son of a medical school president in Massachusetts, drew up a charter for one. A few months later, in the winter of 1837, they had it presented to the legislature in Vandalia, then the state capital.

They named the new school after Benjamin Rush, a Philadelphia physician active in Revolutionary politics and a post-Revolutionary medical and humanitarian leader, who had died in 1813. Rush was the only formally trained physician who signed the Declaration of Independence. The first president, George Washington, was his patient.

Rush pioneered in psychiatry and published papers and books about alcoholism. His theories about "excess excitability" of blood vessels led to a controversial emphasis by him on bleeding and purging of patients. In Philadelphia in 1786, he founded the nation's first free dispensary and later was professor of medicine at the newly founded University of Pennsylvania. His family was well established in Philadelphia, and Brainard hoped to gain financial support from family members.

Goodhue was a prominent civic figure and debater who pushed successfully for the city's first public school system. He died in 1847 when he fell into an open well while making a night house call. Another was Dr. John T. Temple, who like many physicians of the day, had wide business interests. His shipping firm was the first to ship mail out of Chicago. He operated a stagecoach line and built part of the Illinois-Michigan canal. Another of Brainard's contacts, Dr. Edmund S. Kimberley, was a commercial pharmacist who sold patent medicines.

They and Brainard and other incorporators received their charter for Rush Medical College on March 2, 1837, two days before the city of Chicago received its charter. It was the first school of any kind chartered by Illinois, the first health care institution in Chicago, one of the first medical schools west of the Alleghenies. The date was otherwise inauspicious. The year was one of financial panic and depression, and the school's opening had to be delayed. Neither did the Rush family see fit to contribute to its support, as Brainard had hoped. An interim began.

Brainard became the city's first health officer and served for a year. He was appointed to the largely inactive Chicago Board of Health in 1838 and in that year did a difficult leg amputation (for an injured canal worker) with medical colleagues watching. He performed with his usual boldness and coolness and made a reputation that attracted the first of his "aristocratic" clientele.

As a frontier surgeon, he was no bumpkin. His polish set him apart. Indeed, some considered him cold and remote, apparently because of his seriousness and directness. Later, he was the first to use ether in the city, while amputating a finger at the dispensary in Tippecanoe Hall, at Wolcott and Kinzie streets on January 12, 1847. It was the same dispensary where chloroform was used 12 days later—either by Brainard or another surgeon—10 days before it was used in New York.

In 1839 Brainard went to Paris, where he observed and performed various studies, doing a number of surgical procedures on cadavers. He returned to Paris in the mid-1850s and again in 1866, just before he died, each time to revel in the opportunities for experimentation which he found there. He liked it there, and they liked him. The superintendent of the "garden of plants" in Paris, where experimental animals were kept, approved his work and gave him the help he needed.

Brainard was a scientist, unlike most of his medical colleagues in the U.S., where a sort of common sense empiricism was the order of the day. Furthermore, when he wrote about his work, either experimental or surgical, he did it in the context of what others were doing and recording. He weighed and balanced various procedures, carefully noting pros and cons. His article on un-united fractures won a prize.

But he and his colleague James Van Zandt Blaney, whom he met during this interim, were exceptions to the rule. U.S. and especially Midwestern doctors were not systematic experimenters, but rather tried things out at random, pretty much in isolation from each other. Brainard and Blaney were two of the few who pursued solutions with the systematic approach we call science.

One of the factors that worked against experimentation was widespread Midwestern antipathy to dissection of cadavers, which in turn led to the "body-snatching" and grave-robbing problem immortalized by Mark Twain in his *Adventures of Tom Sawyer*. (Tom and Huckleberry Finn watched the murder of a young doctor by one of his grave-robbing accomplices, Injun Joe.) Indeed, medical schools were damned if they did and didn't equally: without cadavers they could not train students in anatomy, with them the public rose up to complain.

A school in St. Charles, Illinois, west of Chicago, broke up when a mob invaded its quarters and shot the president. Years later, in 1857, a Rush student and the city sexton were charged with "resurrectionism" (student's term for body-snatching) and were vilified in the press as "hyenas" and "barbarians." Before 1859 the only bodies available were those of hanging victims, and not until 1885 did Illinois law give students access to paupers' bodies otherwise destined for burial at public expense.

In 1842 Brainard taught at St. Louis University medical

school. The Rush trustees had met at least once while Brainard had been in Paris. As would be the case a hundred years later, the Rush charter was there to be used, but the users had to await their opportunity. In St. Louis Brainard met the young and likable Dr. James Van Zandt Blaney, whom Brainard recruited as the school's first teacher.

In 1843 Brainard finally opened his medical school. (He had given anatomy lessons in the interim, in his office.) In his inaugural address, he set forth noble goals. "The health, the happiness and the life of your dearest friends and your own," he told the students, "may and will some day depend on the skill of some member of the [medical] profession . . . . To elevate the standard of skill and knowledge in the profession, to excite an honorable emulation among its members, to disseminate for their successors in this new region the principles of medical science . . . such are the objects held in view by the founders of this institution."

The institution's curriculum was standard: two 16-week lecture courses, held in the winter so the farm boys wouldn't miss planting or harvesting, of which the second simply repeated the first. There was a variation: the second 16 weeks could be dropped in favor of two years working with "a respectable physician." In any case, three more years were apparently required with such a preceptor. The Doctor of Medicine degree recipient had to be 21 and of good character. He had to present a thesis in his own handwriting for faculty approval, in addition to passing examinations on lectures. Students were male.

The sole female student during Rush's first 60 years or so, Emily Blackwell, was dismissed in 1852 after Rush was censured by the Illinois State Medical Society for accepting her. Students were white except for David Jones Peck, whose Doctor of Medicine degree in 1847 was the first for a U.S. black from a U.S. medical school.

Fees were $10 a course, or $60 a term, plus a $20 graduation fee and $5 to cover dissection costs if the student were so inclined. Fees were payable by note in some cases, but these were not always collectible. When Austin Flint, one of the first

Rush teachers, returned East, he took notes with him; they weren't worth much in Chicago and presumably declined in value the farther east he traveled. Flint said he would not return to Chicago until they were paid. They apparently weren't; he certainly didn't. Board was $2 a week.

Later, Rush teacher Nathan Davis, intent on opening medical education to as many as possible, insisted on reducing fees, which were dropped to $35 a term. Some 20 years later, in 1879, the regular medical schools of Chicago and Cincinnati agreed to fix fees at $75; it was one more step in removing medical education from the category of "a competitive commodity," to use historian Thomas Bonner's phrase.

Twenty-two students matriculated in Rush's first class, in December of 1843. They met for lectures in a rented hall in the Saloon Building on Clark Street south of the river. Teachers and students waded through mud to the minimally furnished classrooms.

Plans were already afoot to build. Civic leaders William B. Ogden, the city's first mayor and chairman of the Rush board, and Walter Newberry and others offered help if Rush moved north, across the Chicago River. This is where the first Rush building went up, at the corner of Dearborn Street and what is now Grand Avenue, in the summer of 1844, at a cost of $3,500, most of it from faculty pockets. The *Chicago Democrat* called it "an ornament to the city." Rush Medical College was showing people that Chicago could hold its head high not only commercially but intellectually and morally as well, the newspaper proclaimed.

Operating expenses were financed in part by sale of stock certificates at $50 each. These were apparently donations or free loans, redeemable at face value but earning no interest for the buyer. Later, in 1855, another building was erected. The faculty again covered the cost. Indeed, Rush trustees (who held bonds that did earn interest) were mostly faculty throughout the century. Rush was not for profit, but it was run as if it were.

This is not to say there was much money to be made from the venture. The problem with the proprietary schools (and most were proprietary) was not profit-taking but control. And in Rush's case, non-proprietary as it may have been, Brainard pretty much ran the show, as became clear when he successfully resisted a faculty majority in the late fifties.

As for Rush's moneymaking potential, it could not have been much. Blaney may have decorated his cabin beyond frontier standards, and Rush professors bought their surgical instruments in Europe, but none of this pointed to their Rush connection as a source of wealth. Medical education in general at the time was a business, it is true, entered mostly for profit by entrepreneurs, including instructors. There was sharp competition for students and low standards, such as eight months "reading" with a practitioner for whom students "ground the powders and mixed the pills." That and four months of listening to lectures, and one had his M.D.

By the start of Rush's third year, in any event, the school enjoyed "increasing facilities," according to the *Chicago Democrat*. By 1848 it had produced 71 graduates, 30 in the class of '48. It had given five honorary degrees.

Teachers were picked for their lecturing ability. Not until the 1880s did lecturing begin to give way in medical schools, and then to periodic student recitation as an aid to motivation, as Nathan Davis urged. These early lecturers were a young lot, as befitted their pivotal roles in a young city, not to mention profession, since medical education was in a pioneer state as well. In Rush's first 16 years, 12 of its 14 professors were 35 or younger. Among the first were James Blaney, William Herrick (no relation to the famous James Herrick, who came later), Austin Flint and Moses Knapp (who was older than 35).

James Van Zandt Blaney was all of 23 when he became a charter member of the Rush faculty, teaching chemistry and pharmacy. An attractive young man of winning disposition, he was much liked by students and about everyone else, for that matter. Without fanfare, as was his style, he started the city's first medical dispensary in his office across the street from the Sherman House, reportedly in 1839. Later, Brainard began a surgical dispensary to go with it, to greater acclaim—

testimony to Brainard's personality as much as the substance of the achievement.

In 1843 the combined medical-surgical dispensary was moved to the newly occupied Rush Medical College building. Its attending physicians were largely Rush faculty. In 1845 it was moved to a large warehouse called Tippecanoe Hall, at Wolcott and Kinzie streets, where Brainard, Blaney and William Herrick established Chicago's first general hospital in 1847. This was the first Cook County hospital, insofar as the county furnished most of its supplies.

But it didn't last long, and dispensaries remained the nearest thing to a hospital. People went either to a doctor's office or a dispensary, which in essence provided outpatient care. At the latter they could pay or not, according to ability. Paying patients might use the dispensary, which was not much publicized; people just seemed to know it was there. It provided no place to keep trauma cases, of course. As such it was prelude to the hospital, which could lodge such patients.

The Rush faculty was extensively involved in organizing hospitals. The first to survive was the Illinois General Hospital of the Lakes, which opened in 1850 in rooms rented at the Lake House Hotel at North Water and Rush streets. This hospital was largely the work of Nathan Davis. Brainard ran surgery, Dr. John Evans ran obstetrics, Davis and Dr. Levi Boone ran the medical department. Medical students did the nursing according to a vague arrangement that proved unsatisfactory. The Sisters of Mercy took over the nursing and running of the place in 1851. The Rush faculty reserved beds in return for its offer of free care to the needy.

As for Blaney, who in a sense started it all with his dispensary, work at the dispensary wasn't enough in the way of extracurriculars. He also was founding editor of *The Illinois Medical and Surgical Journal,* the city's first such publication, in 1844. In its first issue he explained, as does every editor in a maiden issue, that his publication was to meet needs not being met, in this case among Midwest physicians.

It would carry local medical news, including epidemic statistics and descriptions of remedies both reliable and otherwise. The latter would be branded as "newfangled impostures," and

Midwestern doctors and their patients would be suitably warned. The journal, later called the *Chicago Medical Journal* and edited by Rush professors Evans and Davis, ran mostly reprints from Eastern and European publications. Some Rush originals also were printed, including articles by Evans and others on the dreaded cholera. Later it served as a vehicle for one side of the Brainard-Davis feud of the 1860s.

Blaney also lectured around the city to great effect and success, and later succeeded Brainard as president of Rush following Brainard's death in 1866.

William B. Herrick, 31, a Dartmouth M.D., class of 1836, and an Illinoisan since 1839, was a popular anatomy lecturer. Promoted to professor in 1845 in recognition of his popularity with students, but over objections of some of his Rush colleagues, he left not much later for service in the Mexican War. From Mexico he wrote letters to Blaney's journal about health conditions among U.S. troops and in Mexico in general. He returned to teach at Rush, where he remained until 1857. In 1850, he became the first president of the Illinois State Medical Society.

Another of the original faculty, Austin Flint, stayed three years at Rush and then returned east to build a distinguished career as author and professor at Bellevue Hospital Medical College in New York City.

Brainard's evident keen ability to choose top performers stands out even more brightly when one considers the mistakes that were available to him as demonstrated in the case of Moses Knapp. Knapp was not liked by the students and was cashiered at the end of the first 16-week term. Once dismissed, he told stories about his former colleagues apparently to discredit them, leading Blaney to conclude they had been doubly right to fire the man. Then Knapp was caught seeking to lead a young girl astray on graduation night at the La Porte, Indiana, medical school, where he taught after Rush, and was dismissed from that institution as well. Nonetheless, he had in all an apparently distinguished career in and out of Chicago, including a stint as dean of the Rock Island (Illinois) Medical School, which eventually became part of the University of Iowa.

Ferment in Medical Education
1836-1871

The second wave of Rush teachers brought with it the Nestor of Chicago medicine, Dr. Nathan S. Davis, already founder of the American Medical Association and founder-to-be of Northwestern University Medical School. He was also an evangelist and prophet for reform in medical education and was destined to be a thorn in the side of his counterpart at Rush, Daniel Brainard, who, it may be said, gave him his start in Chicago.

Known for his activism in the cause of medicine and medical education, Davis was recruited for Rush at the AMA convention in Boston in 1849 by John Evans, another trailblazer whom Brainard had already drawn to Chicago.

Evans was a mental-health progressive from Indiana, praised by reformer Dorothea Dix for his work in that state on behalf of the mentally ill. A Cincinnati College medical graduate, class of 1838, who overcame his Quaker father's objections to studying medicine, Evans became also a railroad and real estate investor and philanthropist. He played a key role in founding Northwestern University (its location, Evanston, bears his name), took an abolitionist position on slavery and spent the last 36 years of his long life in Colorado, where he began as territorial governor and among other things founded the University of Colorado.

Evans was a gung-ho recruiter for Rush, which he joined in 1844, enthusiastically pumping the hinterlands for students, going in fact beyond what Brainard thought suitable. Brainard didn't believe in pushing young men in the matter of medical careers. He thought Evans overdid it.

Maybe Brainard came to think Evans overdid it when Evans brought the prophetic, reformist Davis into Chicago. Davis's first big splash was to call immediately for free medical education, something he said both community and students deserved, stating this as a Rush goal. On the spot he promised three free "tickets," as they were called, for Rush courses. Other schools naturally complained at the underpricing, but Davis was unmoved. Native ability alone should be the only requirement for medical school, he said. Indeed, he is better known for his insistence on higher requirements, of which more later.

Another of this second wave of Rush teachers was Edmund Andrews, a paragon of the polymath physician. An expert in botany, zoology, ornithology and geology, he pioneered in antisepsis and in 1856 helped found the Chicago Academy of Natural Sciences (of which Blaney was the first president). His adding of oxygen to nitrous oxide made long-term anesthesia safe.

These gentlemen were teaching and practicing medicine and surgery in virtually epidemic surroundings. The state was only decades removed from the "graveyard" category into which it had been lumped early in the century. One Illinois county in the 1820s had lost 80 percent of its population to malaria. In Chicago the chief problem, worse even than malaria and typhus, was cholera, which broke out in 1832 and 1849, providing a number of scares in between.

The city's bad reputation endured into the 1850s. In 1850 it had no sewerage system. Davis pushed for one and in addition lectured on alcoholism, infant care and other matters of personal hygiene. Like Brainard, he stayed abreast of the latest.

"Out of the hydrants came fish dinners. Millions of rats lived under raised wooden walks," said one breezy chronicler years later, when it was too late to count the rats. In this frontier-like town, men far outnumbered women: by three to two in the 20–50 age bracket. Over half the people were foreign-born: 52 percent in contrast to New York's 45 percent.

In the midst of it all stood Rush Medical College, already in 1850 the 10th largest of the nation's 150 medical schools. And within its not yet hallowed walls, a first-class fight was brewing.

Davis had brought with him strong ideas about the ideal availability of medical education. On the one hand he wanted it unrestricted by cost considerations, on the other more rigidly restricted according to ability. He also faced up to the anomaly of the curriculum: the bright students he wanted to attract were asked to sit through two identical 16-week lecture courses.

He pushed immediately, therefore, for a "graded curriculum," that is, one in which the second year built on the first without repeating it, offering clinical matter as follow-up on basic science. Andrews the multifaceted scholar backed him up. They and others pressured the "imperious and autocratic" Brainard, who for various reasons resisted.

Among them was the natural reluctance of the successful to change their ways. The Rush way was how everyone did it. Older students probably took some responsibility for teaching younger ones. The system seemed to be working, illogical as it was. Anyhow, wasn't repetition the mother of studies?

Secondly, good teachers were hard to find. Nobody knew that better than Brainard, who had already put together several faculties. There was the serious question whether doubling the curriculum content might not put a strain on or even exhaust the available teacher-pool. It was the sort of thing a medical school founder who had been there might worry about.

Nonetheless, Brainard found himself a minority of one on the graded-curriculum issue, if not at first, then at least by the summer of 1857, when in his absence the faculty voted in favor of it. The die being thus cast, they told Brainard on his return that they wanted to take it to the trustees. Brainard said no, he would take it. He did and returned with the answer no. Rush would not switch.

If Rush wouldn't, Davis, Andrews and others would. In 1859 they left Rush to form their own school, Chicago Medical College, which later became Northwestern University Medical School. The split was permanent and it was a blow to Rush. Davis and five allies—Hosmer Johnson, William Byford, David Rutter, Ralph Isham, and Andrews—took Mercy Hospital with them, leaving Rush without adequate clinical training facilities. Brainard's students had to use their dispensary and later the U.S. Marine Hospital, neither of which apparently was a match for Mercy.

Brainard, bitter, criticized Davis and the others, though not by name, as "incompetent, noisy individuals." Medical knowledge, he maintained, depended not on curriculum but on teacher. If you wanted to improve it, you got better teachers. Neither did you cut fees, as Davis wanted to do, since fee income paid for better libraries and led to better educated doctors. Brainard's approach was to multiply students, not requirements.

When Davis said the country was full of "half-educated physicians," Brainard called him a traitor to the cause of the "regular" physicians, as opposed to homeopathic and other "irregular" physicians, calling Davis's comment "an unjust attack upon physicians and schools." Davis was no softy on the homeopathic question, however. In 1850, as secretary of Rush Medical College, he had refused admission to a homeopath, that is, a doctor who cured with minute doses of what in large amounts would induce the symptoms.

In drinker's parlance, homeopathy offers a hair of the dog that bit you. In those days it enjoyed considerable popular support, and the dispute between the two schools was a lively one. The allopath, one who sought directly to alleviate symptoms, was classed as "regular," however.

Davis's refusal of the homeopathic applicant had caused a protest over alleged violation of the man's rights. Again, in 1857, he had refused to serve on the staff of the new city hospital because homeopaths would also be serving there. A typical man of principle, Davis was hard to live with at times.

Brainard had his own prickliness. He also refused cooperation when he felt used, as when he led a boycott in 1850 of the newly formed Chicago Medical Society, which elected as president Dr. Levi D. Boone, who later won the Chicago mayoralty on the Know-Nothing ticket. Brainard, who looked on medical societies as "trade unions" concerned with fee standards or "punitive leagues" concerned with ethics enforcement, didn't like Boone anyhow. So the decision was an easy one. His boycott killed the baby society, but Davis, a proven believer in group action, revived it two years later.

Brainard instead gave his support to a rival organization with more professional and academic goals, the Chicago Academy of Medical Sciences, which was founded in 1859 and consisted largely of Rush teachers for its three years' existence.

Meanwhile, Davis announced the program for his new school in an inaugural address at Market (later Wacker) and Randolph streets, in a building called Lind's Block. (His school began under the aegis of the short-lived Lind University. Decades later, Northwestern University took it over.) The program included these changes (or reforms) from the accepted way of doing things: a five-month term (versus 16 weeks), fewer lectures per day, more professors, full recognition of clinical chairs, daily clinical hospital experience for students, and the vaunted graded curriculum. Bonner notes that Harvard did not adopt these changes for 12 years. On the other hand, neither was all of it strange and new, notably the clinical training part, which was a Rush staple from the start.

Rush resisted most of this, waiting nine years to add two weeks to its course length and 17, well after Brainard's death, to adopt the graded curriculum. The Brainard-Rush position was that graded curriculum forced students to cram basics in their first year while neglecting them in the second, clinical, year. In 1868, *The Chicago Medical Journal,* a Rush-allied publication, referred to Davis not complimentarily as "the apostle" and to his school as "the reform school."

The competition did not hurt Rush enrollment, however. It

rose from 119 in 1859, the year Chicago Medical College began, to 374 in 1866, the year of Brainard's death. Chicago Medical College on the other hand did not reach 100 students until 1865. Some of Rush's enrollment gains, it should be noted, came from courses offered in military surgery during the war.

Davis later promoted another reform, higher entrance requirements. As early as 1867, he required English, mathematics, science, Latin and Greek of his incoming students. This sort of thing had no appeal to the Rush administration. Of 135 students in the Rush class of 1888, for instance, only seven had a college diploma of any kind, according to its distinguished alumnus James Herrick, a man of extensive liberal arts credentials in his own right. Only by 1891 did Rush ask applicants to prepare themselves in algebra, geometry, rhetoric, logic, Latin, English and physics—20 years after the state first tried to raise entrance requirements in Illinois medical schools.

In all this Davis comes off the dreamer, Brainard the mossback. But Brainard had his dreams too, in scientific medicine. He had been impressed in Paris with the French emphasis on student involvement in hospital work and experimentation and thought lecturing could be overdone. Davis wanted more lectures, though fewer per day. The problem was, as Brainard knew from experience, where to find the lecturers. Rush for its part had from the beginning offered classes in anatomy (with dissection) and clinics in surgery. Rush students from the start learned about medicine in the dispensary.

Davis thought more in societal terms than Brainard and cared deeply about education, but he wasn't the scientist Brainard was. His articles do not refer to others' positions on the matter he was treating. Brainard's always did. So did those of his colleague (and protégé?) Blaney. Judged in this light, Davis was the plunger, Brainard the thoughtful one who took others' opinions into consideration, but it's only one light, and neither profits from too much thumbnail-sketching.

Brainard was arrogant but very good at some things, judging men, for instance. He picked some top-drawer performers and never worried about the competition this would cause him. Witness the hall of fame he gathered around himself at Rush, including Davis. Then beginning all over when Davis and the others left, he put together another good team.

Another difference between the two was that Brainard favored specialization while Davis didn't, even though his graded curriculum idea seemed to call for it. Brainard hired Edward Holmes, the eye doctor, at the first opportunity. He thought it was wonderful that this young man knew so much about the eye. As a result, Rush had its ophthalmology department (after Brainard's death, in 1869) a year before Chicago Medical College.

Finally, perhaps the crucial difference was that Brainard thought education depended on the teacher and patient contact, almost regardless of the curriculum. Davis, more the theoretician and logician in the matter, seemed to put curriculum first.

In a sense these two giants of early Chicago medical education complemented each other. Their feud may be seen as ferment which led to progress, as another kind leads to wine. In any event, neither threw in his lot, in the final analysis, with a losing proposition. The professional heirs of each can be grateful for that.

Brainard the politician and civic figure was a Chicago type. He tied in with the Democrats early in his Chicago experience. By May 1847, he was serving with William B. Ogden, the city's first mayor and president of the Rush board of trustees from 1843 to 1872, on a committee to help raise money for Irish relief during the potato famine.

In 1858, with the slavery question dominant, he ran for mayor on a pro-choice platform, enjoying the support of "every pimp, every shyster, every blackleg, base men and lewd women," who expended "fiendish energy" on his behalf, according to the *Daily Democratic Press,* which obviously did not support his candidacy.

He sided with national or mainstream Democrats in opposition to the moderate position taken by U.S. Sen. Stephen A. Douglas of Illinois. National Democrats had supported the

Dred Scott decision, but Douglas broke with the administration on a related issue, whether the pro-choice Kansas constitution had been fairly presented to the Kansas electorate. In the ensuing political fallout, Brainard sided with the regulars.

Then Douglas faced Lincoln in the 1858 senatorial election, in the midst of which a phony story surfaced that Douglas owned slaves in Louisiana. Brainard was in the middle of this one. He was the first to be told the story, by a visiting Louisianan named Slidell, and passed it on. Slidell and Brainard eventually denied the accuracy of the report but not until it had made the rounds and damaged the Douglas campaign. Douglas won the election, but Brainard lost his, for mayor.

The war years passed, Brainard made what turned out his final trip to France, and then the end came. He died of galloping cholera, on October 10, 1866, a few hours after he was stricken while working on a lecture about the disease to be given that night. An alderman and another doctor died the same day. Brainard was 54 years old.

Two hundred Rush students panicked when they realized how close they were to the dread disease and voted to adjourn classes until December because of the danger. The faculty talked them out of it. "They of all men should not fly," added *The Tribune* editorially, and the students stayed.

The Rush-Chicago Medical College feud began to fade immediately. Davis even drew up a plan for merging the two schools according to which the Rush course would be expanded to five months and the Rush faculty's "proprietary relationship" to their school would be ended. (Rush operated on a not-for-profit charter, but faculty members held the bonds and were its trustees.) But Davis's reunion plan was never taken seriously. Excitement lay ahead but not yet a merger.

Presbyterian Hospital & Rush Medical College in the Late Nineteenth Century 1871–1898

The Chicago fire of 1871 left thousands homeless and devastated the city's medical facilities, including the four-year-old Rush Medical College building at Dearborn Street and Grand Avenue. Dr. Joseph W. Freer, Rush's new president-elect, found his half-melted microscope stand and various pieces of chemistry apparatus in the rubble.

This was all that remained of Rush as a physical plant. Throughout the city, devastation reigned. Over 200 doctors, including most of the Rush faculty, were without home, office, library, entire practices. Moses Gunn, Brainard's successor as professor of surgery, lost books, office, instruments, anatomical specimens and a huge manuscript. Many students lost everything they owned, with no way to replace it.

Ten-year-old James Herrick watched the flames from his home in Oak Park. After the fire his father with other Oak Parkers, including author Ernest Hemingway's grandfather, brought food and blankets to the homeless and hungry, returning shaken from the expedition.

"They were starving," the senior Herrick reported on his

return. Men, women and children, huddled on the Lake Michigan shore, wept and kissed his hand as he distributed sandwiches, crackers, hard-boiled eggs, milk and coffee from his covered delivery wagon. He wept himself as he told of the scene, unable to continue his account.

Later James Herrick rode with his father through the burned-out area, less impressed with the ruins than with the huge unpainted barracks hastily erected by General Phil Sheridan's soldiers to house the homeless during the coming winter. These and soldiers' tents stayed with the memory of the boy who decades later would make his own contribution to the relief of human suffering.

Rush Medical College needed space. Its sole rival, Chicago Medical College (later the Northwestern University Medical School), had escaped the fire. Its leaders, the reformer Davis among them, invited Rush students to continue studies there, at 26th Street and Prairie Avenue, free of charge. Rush did use their dissecting laboratory. But for lecture purposes (and this was the heart of the curriculum), Rush reopened four days after the fire in the small amphitheater on the top floor of Cook County Hospital, at 18th and LaSalle (then Arnold) streets, also on the South Side.

The institution was a "large brick building of a dirty red color . . . in a badly kept lot," with nothing about it to "cheer the spirits of a sick man," according to a news account. Surrounded by a tilting "low, rickety fence," it was neighbor to shanties. The grounds were strewn with garbage. The street was muddy and full of holes. The building was terribly overcrowded.

It was next to this less than salubrious institution and onto these garbage-strewn grounds that Rush moved after the fire. Rush was already almost umbilically tied to this now-County Hospital, which for 11 years had been where its students received the bulk of their clinical training. But Rush College itself had been on the other side of town, three miles north. So the move to the hospital, though forced by catastrophe, nonetheless made sense. Once winter was past, therefore, Rush built on its grounds, partly below sidewalk level. The new building cost $3,500, which was all the trustees could afford.

It was "a rude, brick affair" with a tar roof. On its first floor at one end was an amphitheatre, at the other was a laboratory. Over the lab was a dissecting room. The whole was unplastered throughout and was "very rough and amazingly ugly," Rush historians Norman Bridge, M.D., and John Edwin Rhodes, M.D., tell us. But for under $4,000, Rush students and faculty couldn't complain. The "rude structure," known also as "the college under the sidewalk," served for four years, until both Rush and County Hospital moved to the West Side.

Meanwhile, James V. Z. Blaney, whom Brainard had recruited to the first Rush faculty, retired as president not six years after succeeding the deceased founder. He was 52 and had been in Chicago for almost 30 years after graduating from Princeton and obtaining his M.D. in Philadelphia. He had served as surgeon with the rank of major of artillery during the "war of rebellion," as the Rush yearbook called it. Blaney died two years later.

In 1876, both County Hospital and Rush built anew, this time on the West Side. Rush built on the northeast corner of Harrison and Wood, where a successor building remains; Cook County Hospital built on the southwest corner, where the 1876 structure remains today.

The Rush building was a considerably grander affair than the "rude structure," though Bridge and Rhodes later found it surprising that its anatomy museum, which the students didn't even use, took up more than half its space. The building and lot cost $75,000, mostly contributed by several faculty members who purchased long-term bonds to finance construction.

At cornerstone-laying on March 20, 1875, Grand Master (later Mayor) DeWitt C. Cregier led Masonic ceremonies after a procession of dignitaries, faculty and students, in that order, from the LaSalle Street site. "A great concourse of people" gathered to hear Dr. J. Adams Allen deliver "sonorous periods" which Bridge and Rhodes could compare only to Tennyson reading his own poetry. "Modern Rome is built upon the roofs of its ancient temples and palaces," began

Allen, and took it from there with a historical overview of kingdoms rising and falling.

Ten months later, in January of 1876, Allen gave the first lecture in the finished building, dipping frequently into his "fund of classical lore" to illustrate his remarks.

The destinies of the two neighbor institutions, Rush and County Hospital, were intertwined. Rush had its need for clinical education which County seemed to fill; County had reason to welcome Rush, with its wealth of talent. The relationship would have worked wonderfully if it hadn't depended on people.

At stake was control of this publicly funded hospital, built by the city in 1857 but not opened until it was leased by Rush in 1859. Two doctors who joined the Rush faculty in 1860, Dr. Joseph Presley Ross and Dr. George K. Amerman, apparently had a vision of a public hospital that would meet the health care needs of poor people and the medical education needs of Rush students.

This city-built public hospital was operated by Rush faculty on contract with city government from 1859 to 1862, when the Army took it over. After the war, the issue again lay before Ross and Amerman how to get this public hospital functioning in answer to community needs for health care and medical education. Their solution was to go political. Each got himself elected to the county board of supervisors, Amerman in 1865 and Ross in 1866. Together, they persuaded Cook County authorities to take over. Thus was established Cook County Hospital as such.

Medical politics had to be observed in its organization. Its medical board was to be one part Rush, one part Chicago Medical College (both equal parts), and one part independent (greater than the other two combined)—consisting of doctors connected with neither school.

The arrangement respected medical politics but did not protect against them. In 1867 Dr. Edwin Powell, a newly appointed Rush professor who was also a nephew of the late Brainard, resigned from Rush long enough to be elected to the delicately balanced hospital medical board as an independent. He was then promptly re-elected to the Rush faculty, thus upsetting the delicate balance.

His maneuverings somehow led, four years later, to the dismissal by the county board of the medical board and subsequent increased involvement by politicians in the hospital's affairs. This ended hopes for a self-perpetuating, self-governing medical staff and created an opening for political interference and mismanagement. Control by politicians thus followed on doctors' inability to manage their own affairs.

Rush's clinical education needs were being met in part by its own dispensary, the U.S. Marine Hospital and St. Joseph's Hospital. But County Hospital with its 130 beds (later 750) was the biggest in the city, and it was the basket into which Rush was prepared to put by far the majority of its clinical-training eggs.

So much the more disappointing were developments of the early and middle 1870s, when the County Hospital situation unravelled and the Rush people saw their plans go awry. The culmination of this unravelling process was the mass dismissal by the county board of the medical staff in 1878, an episode shrouded in mystery as far as historical accounts go, its narrative reduced to laconic references to ''disruption'' and reappointment of a new staff.

Whatever the specifics, it was clear to the Rush people that County Hospital would not meet their needs. In 1877 Ross and his allies had seen trouble coming and had already decided Rush should start its own hospital. It would not be the first time the college had done so. Mercy Hospital had begun as the Illinois General Hospital of the Lakes in 1850, largely a Rush faculty creation. Blaney and Brainard had started dispensaries and a short-lived city hospital even before that.

The interest was there from the medical school point of view. As the Rush yearbook of 1895 says, ''The value of clinical instruction can hardly be exaggerated. It far over-shadows didactic lectures and in some institutions has entirely supplanted them.'' Or in the words of the 1894 yearbook,

"Medicine cannot be taught in the abstract; theory without practice is like swimming on dry land." Rush needed a hospital it could control, so that the hospital's service could keep pace with Rush's "didactics."

In 1879, the Rush trustees bought land with the intent to finance and maintain a hospital on their own, but found the challenge more than they could handle. Ross, the faculty's "financial wheelhorse," devised a plan whereby a separate corporation would receive this land in return for Rush control over the planned hospital.

An offer was made on the spot by "a religious body famed for its hospitals and amply able to redeem its pledges," the 1894 yearbook tells us. (Moses Gunn was negotiating with several Catholic nuns' groups.) But Ross, a dedicated Presbyterian, saw no reason why the city's Presbyterian churches could not meet the challenge, as they had done in the case of New York City's Presbyterian Hospital.

To his aid in this venture came several clergy and laymen, including his father-in-law, Tuthill King, who donated $10,000. Others who helped and with King became incorporators of the new institution (on July 21, 1883) were William Blair, Cyrus H. McCormick, Rev. Willis Craig, Henry Lyman and Dr. Robert C. Hamill, after whom was named the 40-bed "Hamill Wing," the hospital's first addition.

The new hospital was chartered to offer "surgical and medical aid and nursing to sick and disabled persons of every creed, nationality and color." At the same time, it was to provide care for the "hundreds of people of the better class" who each year were "stricken by disease or injury," according to an 1883 appeal for funds. The appeal noted that the city's only Protestant general hospital, St. Luke's, was "trying to meet this want" but could "accommodate only a small part of those who apply for hospital care and treatment."

The new Presbyterian Hospital of Chicago opened in September of 1884, with a nominal capacity of 80 beds, 35 of which were needed to house nurses and hospital staff. This first building was the "Ross Wing," named after its chief founder. The Hamill Wing was added a few years later, followed by the 300-bed Daniel A. Jones Memorial Building in 1889.

Jones was a meatpacker, banker, cable car line operator, insurance executive and president of the Chamber of Commerce and the Board of Trade who died a millionaire in 1886. His widow and family gave $100,000 to the hospital, which with $50,000 given by the hospital's president, Dr. D. K. Pearsons, paid for the new building. Jones had already given $10,000 to the hospital, reportedly after reading about the first of Pearsons' gifts, which were spread over several years.

Later additions to the hospital included the Private Pavilion adjoining Jones to the east in 1908 and the Jane Murdock Memorial for women and children in 1912, which to a degree replaced the original Ross and Hamill wings.

On hand for the Murdock building ribbon-cutting ceremonies was Elizabeth Douglass, who later as Mrs. Clyde E. Shorey was for many years to be a mainstay of the hospital's woman's auxiliary. Mrs. Shorey's father, William Angus Douglass, was a member of the founding board of managers and its secretary for more than fifty years.

From the start this auxiliary, or Ladies Aid Society as it was known, gave the hospital crucial support. Consisting of 82 women, including many of Chicago's "leading women," from 17 Presbyterian churches, the society supplied the new hospital with bedding and other linen, kitchenware, utensils and housekeeping appliances. The women supplied patients with various delicacies, books, papers, magazines, even pictures for the walls. They bought "screens, wheelchairs, complete dining room furniture, china, cases of dishes." They read to patients, provided hymn books for Sunday afternoon services and did "much to make the stay of the sick pleasant," according to the second (May 1885) annual report of the hospital.

The Ladies Aid Society became the Woman's Auxiliary Board in 1910. By 1913 it had 200 members. In 1915, membership was opened to non-Presbyterians. In the mid-1920s the Woman's Auxiliary Board recognized "delegate members" whose task was to rally support in the local congregations. In 1928 the name was shortened to Woman's Board, the present name. By the mid-1950s, at the time of the Presbyterian Hospital merger with St. Luke's Hospital, the Woman's Board numbered almost 400 members from 53 Presbyterian churches. Pastors' wives were members ex officio.

The churches for their part began in 1884 to endow annual free beds at $300 each per year, and individuals followed suit. Barbara Armour endowed one in perpetuity for $5,000, Henry Corwith's daughter endowed another for $10,000, and Mrs. William Armour endowed a 10 bed ward for $50,000. The young institution was off to a good start, having tapped an ample philanthropic lode.

Meanwhile, Rush Medical College moved ahead with its clinical education, for which in part it now depended on the new Presbyterian Hospital. Among the early teachers in this new Rush-Presbyterian situation was Dr. Joseph P. Ross himself. A professor of diseases of the chest, Ross was recalled by his student James Herrick as "a good family doctor" who relied heavily on his stethoscope, which he had learned to use from Austin Flint, one of the first Rush teachers (though Ross was not a Rush graduate). He was not highly regarded as a scientist or scholar, however. "Gentlemen," his students would say, mimicking him, "we will now discuss the pathology of tuberculosis. There are two kinds of tubercle, the gray and the yellow. We now pass on to the symptomology of the disease."

Ross is one of those whom Herrick classes as "less scholarly" faculty members, along with William Byford, Moses Gunn, Charles Parkes and James Etheridge, who were nonetheless "earnest, forceful and always understandable," men trained largely by experience, with common sense and an understanding of the needs of undergraduates.

Gunn's surgical clinic drew on his Civil War experience in emergency bone-setting and on his extensive private practice. Having begun his work in the days before anesthesia, he was used to working fast. Herrick saw him repair a child's harelip in five minutes without anesthetic. Gunn withheld judgment on the germ theory, referring to microbes as "little devils," but soaked sutures in carbolic acid solution because he knew it speeded healing.

He was almost never late for lectures and clinics but was held up once by a Chicago River bridge-raising. "Damn the Chicago river bridges," he hurled at a student at the door as he arrived two minutes late. "They are no respecters of college teachers." To the class he apologized, saying he had lost not two minutes of his time but "two minutes' time of each one of you three hundred men," which made 600 minutes, or ten hours. "It was a new point of view," commented Herrick.

A student passed a note to him asking how he kept his hair so curly and who was his barber. Gunn read it aloud and explained how his wife curled his hair every morning, had done so since they were married, and "by the Eternal" would continue to do it as long as she wished. The students loved it.

But when they booed the appearance of a woman intern, Dr. Alta Mitchell, he excoriated them for acting like "Halsted Street hoodlums." Dr. Mitchell was the niece of a good friend of his, Gunn told them. She was competent "and a lady." He had appointed her intern, "and Gentlemen, she's going to stay," he told them. They, however, would leave, all 300 of them, if they booed her again. "Make your choice," he said. They kept quiet and stayed, and so did Dr. Mitchell, who as daughter of the late pastor of First Presbyterian Church had been admitted as an intern "out of respect to her father, though her qualifications eminently fitted her for the place," according to the 1894 yearbook.

Gunn died of cancer in 1887. He was succeeded by Charles T. Parkes, another surgeon of the old school who nonetheless sought younger men's opinions to stay abreast of new discoveries. Parkes was criticized for operating in the clinic on abdominal cases because of the supposed danger of germs dropping into the exposed area—a view on its way to being discredited. He responded: "Gentlemen, I do not know much about these new germs, but I am convinced that what does the harm is not something that may float in the air and settle into the open abdomen. . . . It is what I put into the abdomen that makes the trouble." Therefore he washed and scrubbed his hands and boiled the instruments, gauze and ligatures, going far beyond what his colleagues did in this matter.

Parkes, the first surgeon in the Midwest to experiment in gunshot wounds of the small intestines, died of pneumonia in 1891 at forty-nine. Herrick says he had "a majestic, magnetic personality" and would have been "one of America's outstanding surgeons."

The germ question was central to medical controversies of the day. Antisepsis, the philosophy and procedures by which the surgeon and others fought germs as the cause of disease and infection, was resisted in the 1870s and 1880s even by some heroes of the '50s and '60s. The great Nathan Davis, for instance, in 1876 attacked the notion that specific germs caused specific diseases, arguing that not everyone exposed to them caught the disease in question. He wouldn't accept the argument regarding natural immunity. In 1879 he opposed the imposition of quarantine during an epidemic, still resisting the germ theory.

Moses Gunn, Chicago's best-known surgeon in the 1870s, came around to the new view slowly if at all (opinions differed), holding long to the doctrine of "laudable pus" as a measure of surgical success. Even when he wavered from that view, he still saw suppuration as "a dangerous thorn, from which occasionally, at least, a fragrant flower was plucked."

He had company in his footdragging. In 1883, most surgeons at a meeting in Cincinnati of the American Surgical Association, Gunn among them, agreed with a speaker who deplored the "reckless abandonment" of bloodletting (leeching) in combating inflammation.

Rush had all kinds. James Herrick mentions scholars and old-schoolers and makes it clear he benefited from both. Among the scholars was the immensely learned Dr. Henry M. Lyman, who held the chairs of both physiology, an elementary subject, and neurology, an advanced one. It was a situation that epitomized Rush academic disarray in the mid-1880s. From September to Christmas, Lyman lectured on physiology, from Christmas to late February on neurology. The final examination was on both together. It was not the ultimate in academic good order.

In February of 1887, Lyman, smarting from allegations of

being an easy grader, threw his students two curve balls—two barely defined essay questions, including one about poliomyelitis, a term known to few. Herrick heard a fellow test-taker whisper "infantile paralysis"; so he caught the drift and was one of four who passed out of 200 or so.

Lyman distinguished himself as a neurologist and in 1893 was elected president of the American Neurological Association—the first Chicagoan to hold the position since pioneer neurologist James S. Jewell, of Chicago Medical College, held it in the 1870s.

If the Rush system didn't always make sense, it must be viewed in the context of how little was expected of medical students at the time, and also with a look at the role of the clinics, where students sometimes seemingly through osmosis captured the essence of what had to be known from remarks by the professor.

Not that the students as a rule were hankering for more. Herrick himself, later a major scientific medical figure of his day, had never heard of Rush but was sent there by an Oak Park physician alumnus. He had taught school and considered a career in literary scholarship. When he got to Rush, he found a mixed bag of fellow students. Many were born leaders, bound to succeed in anything they tried. Some of the older ones, veterans of careers as druggists or salesmen or even cowboys, seemed "crude and raw" but had the advantage of beginning with a good working knowledge of human nature. The faculty made the difference, thus confirming Brainard's position some decades earlier in the graded-curriculum controversy.

The students could be a rowdy bunch when the spirit moved them. On one occasion they greeted Lyman with a stunning pre-lecture mess of thrown snowballs, spitballs, overshoes, apples and the like. Lyman entered, and the throwing stopped, but its evidence was there. The arena floor was a pigsty. Lyman turned and walked out, disgusted. There was no lecture that day.

Sometimes the play was vocal, as when three or four hundred voices burst forth at intermission time with "Clementine" or "My Old Kentucky Home." Sometimes it was physical, as in "passing up," when a front-row student was passed bodily up to the last (top) row, where, when he was dropped, the several hundred students stamped their feet as one.

There were free-lance efforts as well. One student, acting as clinical assistant during an operation, took exception to being asked to step aside by another who wanted to see better and thereupon with surgical clamps pulled the other's mustache. The mustached student waited till the operation was over and then punched the other in the nose. "I got what was coming to me, Professor," the punched one explained to Dr. Parkes, the operating surgeon, who took him into the hospital to have his nose fixed.

Other professors whom Herrick considered scholars were Walter S. Haines the chemistry professor, Edward L. Holmes the ophthalmologist, De Laskie Miller the obstetrician, and James Nevins Hyde the dermatologist and author in 1883 of the textbook, *Diseases of the Skin.* A dapper man, Hyde was widely known for his book and for his clinics.

At County Hospital Norman Bridge was one of four attending physicians whom a young doctor was lucky to work under; the others were Christian Fenger, John B. Murphy and P. J. Rowan. His lectures on pathology were considered sound and thorough, however much students chafed at their length.

Compared to Dr. William Quine at the nearby College of Physicians and Surgeons, Bridge was maddeningly vague about the symptoms of typhoid fever. Quine's students got a picture clear as glass but, as students discovered later, somewhat clearer than reality. Diagnosing typhoid was apparently not as easy as a student of Quine might have thought.

Bridge's manner with a patient during clinic was respectful and courteous, even if the patient was poor and ignorant. His diagnosis, furthermore, respected the "natural tendency toward recovery" which called sometimes for "drugless management" of an illness.

One day Bridge informed Herrick that the tuberculosis bacilli he had been examining were Bridge's own—a flareup of an old problem. "In a few days I shall be leaving Chicago never to return," Bridge said matter-of-factly. And he did leave the Chicago medical scene, moving to California for his health. Eventually he made a great deal of money in oil and donated generous amounts to Rush and The University of Chicago. He died at a ripe 81 in 1925.

A "learned and wise medical philosopher," though not a scientist, was Dr. J. Adams Allen, who came to Rush in 1859 as professor of medicine and was Rush's president from 1877 to 1891. Patriarchal in appearance, "Uncle Allen," as he was called, discussed general causes of disease, including temperament or humors or even the weather, rather than symptoms, diagnosis or treatment. He rejected bacteriology and even mocked the stethoscope as just another appurtenance of the pompous diagnostician.

His lectures were scholarly and witty, his anecdotes not always of "the parlor variety." Not surprisingly, he clung to the lecture method and to the large amphitheatre clinic—the sort Will Mayo called "windy (and) wordy"—and routinely recommended consideration of "condition of blood, of the nerve and the part," as students inscribed on a pedestal in his honor. It was not a bad short statement of what caused disease, Herrick noted. Allen died of cancer in 1899.

Dr. De Laskie Miller, who held the Rush chair of obstetrics for many years, was a superb lecturer to whom students listened attentively, without the show of rowdyism that some lecturers inspired. Miller spoke without notes or props, "with exceptional clarity," calling on his wide reading and extensive experience in midwifery.

His successor, J. Suydam Knox, on the other hand, lectured in "casual, rambling" fashion, drawing exclusively on his experience, "of which he often boasted," rather than on scholarship bolstered by practice. In 1892, pediatrics was separated from obstetrics at Rush, with Alfred C. Cotton, a descendant of New England Cottons, its first professor.

"Uncle" Allen's successor as Rush's president was Edward Lorenzo Holmes, the famed ophthalmologist, a Chicagoan since 1856 and principal founder, in 1858, of the Illinois Charitable Eye and Ear Infirmary. As a young man he enjoyed the company of New England literary lights, including the poet Henry Wadsworth Longfellow, and spent summers at the utopian Brook Farm community in Massachusetts. A Harvard College graduate before studying medicine in Vienna, Paris and Berlin, Holmes was a modest and retiring soul. He is said to have been so stunned by the (apparently normal) students' noise and uproar that greeted him when he arrived to give his first lecture at Rush that he turned around and left without lecturing.

William H. Byford, one who had left Rush with Nathan Davis to start Chicago Medical College in 1859 and later had been founding president of Woman's Medical College, lectured in gynecology at Rush in the mid-1880s, having rejoined Rush in 1879. Always on time for class, dignified, deliberate, he began each lecture session by quizzing students, calling names from a class list. He spoke without notes—"plain, straightforward talks" without repetition. When the bell rang, he stopped, bowed politely, took his hat and left. Byford died in 1890, apparently of angina pectoris.

By the 1890s the Rush yearbook was claiming the biggest surgical clinic in the world, as to numbers of students and cases, thanks to the Presbyterian Hospital connection. On the minds of clinic students sometimes overflowing the 300-seat college amphitheatre were "photographed lasting impressions of great value." At Rush "the limited value of didactic work" was recognized. Indeed, the gynecological and medical clinics and the clinics in eye and ear, chest and throat, skin and venereal and children's diseases "afforded unsurpassed opportunity" to graduate and undergraduate students.

Professor Nicholas Senn's surgical clinic met on Tuesdays from 2 to 4 and Thursdays from 2 to 6. They were "the greatest in the world," said the yearbook. Cleanliness "in the strict modern sense" was "the watchword." In the first hour, recent patients were presented as sequel to preceding clinics and as sample of results achieved. A student "consulting staff" was subjected to the "ordeal" of Senn's cross-examination. During operations Senn himself gave a running account.

The Swiss-born Senn, raised in Wisconsin, was one of the Big Three in Chicago surgery in the late 19th and early 20th centuries, with Christian Fenger and John B. Murphy (Fenger's student). An 1868 Chicago Medical College graduate who had studied in Munich, Senn joined the Rush faculty in 1878 as professor of surgery after practicing in Chicago at County Hospital and in Milwaukee. He combined American practicality with German analytical methods and was a top diagnostician though not as good a teacher as Fenger, according to a former student writing in 1896.

Courageous, brilliant and original, he once planted cancer in his arm in an experiment which if successful would have ended his life. A hard worker with "a passion for authorship" and an encyclopedic memory, he was inclined to hasty judgments to which he clung tenaciously. "To be on good terms with him," wrote William Quine in 1908, "you could not question his supremacy." Those who managed to show proper respect, however, found him "a prodigy of generosity" and a delight to be with.

One of Senn's research areas was gunshot wounds. Many years after his death, Dr. Francis Straus found a room in the basement of the old Rush building filled with guns, including a "Nadel Gewehr" from the German army of the 1850s. Senn worked with animals, shooting them in the abdomen which he then explored in order to find and close the bullet holes. His assistant would bubble hydrogen through a catheter into the animal's rear and then light matches (!) to find the leaks. Senn toured Europe demonstrating this technique.

Senn's contemporary, who in some ways overshadowed him and like him had a Chicago high school named after him, was Christian Fenger, a Danish-born surgeon and pathologist who arrived in Chicago from Egypt in 1877. (Chicago elementary schools are also named after Rush teachers Norman Bridge, William Byford, Nathan Davis and John B. Murphy and after alumnus Frank Reilly.) Fenger had worked directly for the Khedive, or Egyptian ruler, who had rewarded him for research on trachoma in part by the gift of several mummy heads. The story is told that he brought an entire mummy with him and sold it to make ends meet in his first months in Chicago; but his daughter, Augusta Marie Fenger Nadler, of Winnetka, said there was no record of any such large baggage or transaction.

His early days in Chicago were financially difficult, however. Before going to Egypt, the young Fenger had studied in Copenhagen and served in two wars. Like Senn, he made gunshot wounds a specialty. He then went off to Vienna to study surgery and pathology, returning to Copenhagen, where in one year he did 422 postmortems. Failing to win an important university appointment when a competitive examination was not given, he left for Egypt, whence he came to the U.S. after two years.

Sick and almost out of money when he arrived in Chicago, he began a small practice and in the spring of 1878, with the help of a Danish-born merchant, bought himself an appointment to the politically controlled County Hospital. He was a lecturer and demonstrator in pathology, which was unknown territory for his listeners, and filled in for other surgeons when they went on vacation. In 1879 he took a one-year appointment at Rush as lecturer in pathological anatomy. In 1880 he was appointed to the regular surgical staff at County and at the same time became "curator" of the Rush "museum" of pathology specimens.

He had arrived at County a "stammering Dutchman." (He could stammer in seven languages, it was said of him.) W. E. Quine asked him to do an autopsy and was given "one of the most astounding experiences" of his life as he watched Fenger at work. Later he told a student that this "Dutchman," the Danish Fenger, would be "Chicago's greatest surgeon." Students flocked to watch him. He was the best they had seen at translating autopsy findings into clinical terms and assumed legendary proportions as a diagnostician.

For his clinics at County, he was at first given the second half of a two-hour lunch period. Among the few at the start who came to view and help were L. L. McArthur and J. B. Murphy, who were smart enough to know what they would otherwise be missing. "Fascinated" by Fenger's technique and "thrilled" by his findings, the two were the vanguard of hundreds who learned pathology from Fenger, who came to be regarded by interns as a court of last resort in difficult cases.

Before performing major surgery he would read on the subject in several languages, summarizing it all the night before and outlining it the next day on a blackboard for his students, listing seventeen steps to the removal of a bronchial cyst, for instance. Sometimes he would stop in the middle of an operation, cover the wound and go to the blackboard to sketch what was happening. Now and then, absorbed in his subject, he would forget to wash his hands as he returned to the patient, and students would intercept him on his way back to the operating table.

His operations took longer than normal for the time, up to six hours. Indeed, he was considered "too thorough for the abdomen" by his onetime clinical assistant, Dr. T. A. Davis, closing off every nook and cranny that might be host to suppuration or bleeding. His student Murphy, on the other hand, "got in and out" as fast as he could. During one period Murphy performed twenty-three appendectomies without a fatality, while Fenger with his thoroughness and slowness considered 50 percent a good record.

He once performed a thyroidectomy with *Gray's Anatomy* on one easel and his own drawings from Swiss surgeon Emil Theodor Kocher on another, having an assistant turn the pages of each as various muscles and the like came into view. At one point he rather roughly handled (with forceps) a laryngeal nerve, picking off bits of thyroid or fat until it lay exposed, at which point he said, "There, now I know where it is and that I have not cut it."

Next morning he checked with the patient, a 35-year-old woman, and asked her to sing, then to say "Ah." She did so, whispering hoarsely, and Fenger, knowing he had handled the nerve too roughly, said, "God damn it to hell" and walked out. It was his expression of guilt at being too thorough in handling and exposing the nerve. The woman did not suffer permanent damage to voice or health, however.

On another occasion he cancelled a 9 A.M. operation at 7:30. He told his helper Herrick about it but not the patient, nurses, relatives and friends. At 10:30 Fenger walked in and explained briefly to the dozen or so waiting people why he had decided not to perform the operation. He left most of the explaining to Herrick, however, leaving abruptly with his bag of instruments. The autopsy later showed that Fenger was correct, the operation would have been useless.

In this performance Fenger demonstrated his "childlike lack of tact" but also perhaps his shrewdness and understanding of human nature, Herrick says. In any event it was typical of both his thoroughness and his honesty.

Fenger died of pneumonia in 1902, a few days after his last clinic, in which he performed a laryngectomy. The operation finished, he went behind a screen to change his clothes while his assistants dressed the wound. But in a minute he was back in front of his students, dressed only in long underdrawers, bare from the waist up, to make a small point he had missed. It was about 6:30 P.M., and all but a few students had left. That night at 2 A.M. he had a chill, developed lobar pneumonia, and several days later was dead.

Fenger's achievement was to draw the connection between pathology and surgery for Chicago doctors. Before him the paths of pathologist and surgeon did not cross, the surgeon being more interested in results than in knowing why he got them. He introduced surgical pathology as a basis for surgical therapy.

Another lecturer in pathology at Rush at this time was William T. Belfield, who promoted acceptance of the new science of bacteriology by showing lantern slides of microorganisms. In 1883 Belfield did an autopsy on a tuberculosis victim, inviting his audience to come down from their Rush amphitheatre seats and look through the microscope at the bacillus he uncovered. But there was no systematic teaching of bacteriology at Rush until 1896, when Edwin C. Klebs, the famous German investigator of typhoid fever and diptheria, assumed the chair of bacteriology and Rush became the center of attention in this new field.

Belfield endorsed the ideas of Robert Koch, the founder of bacteriology, calling them no mere theory but an "ocular demonstration" of germs as the cause of tuberculosis. His published lectures on the relationship between bacteria and disease at the College of Physicians & Surgeons in New York comprise one of the earliest U.S. sources on bacteriology.

Another promoter of Koch's views was Frank Billings, who returned from Vienna in 1886 bringing urine tests, instruments and slides which he explained to his students at the Northwestern University–affiliated Chicago Medical College (finally united with the university in 1891). Billings' distinguished career at Rush was to begin some years later, in 1898.

One of Fenger's prime successors in pathology in Chicago, Ludvig Hektoen, joined the Rush faculty in 1890 as curator of its "museum" of pathology specimens and lecturer in pathological anatomy and histology. He had interned in pathology under Fenger at County Hospital and may have participated in the Wednesday night sessions at Fenger's apartment on Ohio Street, to which came "students and doctors of all ages" to pore with him over slides viewed under microscope.

In 1890 Hektoen also became Chicago's first coroner's physician. Later he was County Hospital pathologist and headed the McCormick Institute for Infectious Diseases, which was eventually renamed after him.

The County Hospital internship was a prize won by a disproportionate number of Rush graduates between 1887 and 1894—66 of 147. Rush, in fact, was one of four medical schools which prepped students for the competitive examination.

Herrick and Hektoen were interns together at County for eighteen months beginning in April of 1888. Herrick joined the Rush faculty in 1889 as assistant demonstrator of anatomy, a year later added a lecturing position on materia medica, and in 1891 became an adjunct professor of medicine. The two were to loom big in the life of Rush during its next phase, the years of its connection to The University of Chicago.

Another affiliation preceded that one, however—with Lake Forest University from 1887 to 1898. The affiliation was nominal and existed for purposes that were vague on both sides. Lake Forest University, in the distant north suburb of that name, had all of 63 students and 13 teachers, compared to Rush's 392 students and 35 teachers. The university title was questionable at best.

What was in it for Lake Forest was the possibility of control of a major institution that dwarfed it. The Lake Forest endowments would accrue to Rush until Rush's debts were retired, at which time ownership of Rush would revert to Lake Forest. What was in it for Rush was the possibility of substantial financial aid without loss of academic autonomy, which the agreement guaranteed.

The "curious" agreement was struck on June 21, 1887. But the affiliation in the end was advantageous to neither party. The hope on which it was based, that Lake Forest would gain a medical school while Rush gained financial independence, never materialized. By 1897 Rush was the biggest medical school in the U.S., with 848 students and 80 teachers, and money was no longer the problem it had been 10 years earlier, such were the student fees such a student body generated.

Meanwhile, the two institutions functioned worlds apart. The Rush baseball team got probably as close as any Rush entity to Lake Forest, defeating its nominal affiliate 17–1 in 1894. This was the year Rush footballers tied Notre Dame 6–6. Few Lake Forest students moved on to Rush for the Doctor of Medicine degree, as the Lake Forest leadership hoped would happen. Rush was doing rather nicely in a money way. Late in 1897 the end of the affiliation drew near.

Doctors De Laskie Miller and Henry Lyman and Trustee Nathan M. Freer were authorized to discuss the matter with the Lake Forest president and board. They discovered the two boards' feelings were mutual, and the relationship was dissolved in June of 1898.

St. Luke's Hospital
is Established
1864–1900

Chicago was "a pretty crude place" when St. Luke's Hospital was founded in 1864 by the Reverend Clinton Locke, rector of Grace Episcopal Church at Peck Court (later 8th Street) and Wabash Avenue. Catholics operated "a small but excellent pay hospital," Locke notes in his memoirs. The only other was the City Free Hospital at 18th and Arnold (later La Salle) streets, "a small, dirty, ill-arranged place, devoid of all comfort."

Locke's own church was nothing to write home about to the folks back in his native Sing Sing (later Ossining), N.Y. It was the same "hideous wooden building" he had discovered five years earlier when he had arrived from Joliet—"a wretchedly built, run-down wooden shell, scattered and peeled."

Some of this was simply life in the big city. In due time Locke had a new church and lived in what he considered ease and comfort. But some of it, such as that City Free Hospital, was bad by any standard. One night he returned from visiting a patient there in a bug-infested room and decided to do something about it. He was inspired, he was "not afraid to say, by the spirit of God."

A week or two later he preached about the need for "a clean, free, Christian place where the sick poor might be cared for." Among his listeners were women of the parish already committed to helping the sick—members of the Camp Douglas Ladies Aid Society, who cared for sick Confederate prisoners held at 33rd Street and Cottage Grove Avenue.

They came to him after the service, his wife Adele at their head, and asked why there shouldn't be a "church hospital." And would he take the lead in starting one? It was an answer to Locke's sermon and to the "whisper" in his soul.

On the next day, February 18, 1864, Locke met with the Douglas society women at the F. B. Hadduck house. They made him president of the new hospital. Dr. Walter Hay became its first doctor. Neither the women nor Locke knew anything about running a hospital, but they were willing to learn. They went to work not in "rising to a point of order," or "moving to adjourn," or "laying a motion on the table, as so many of their daughters and granddaughters" were doing 30 years later, when Locke wrote his memoirs. "They just worked as hard as they could to get the hospital going."

They raised $1,500 and "comfortably furnished" a small wooden house on State Street near Eldridge Court (later East Ninth Street), "a pleasant little place with grass and flowers and one or two poplar trees." Into it they crowded seven beds. Two nurses cared for patients. The first patient, a delirium tremens victim, left unguarded for a moment, jumped out a window, seized a knife from a butcher shop and stabbed a pedestrian, who presumably became the next patient.

Another early patient, ostensibly paralyzed, recovered rapidly when the skeptical Hay instructed a nurse in the patient's presence to prepare a hot poker for some cauterizing of the spine the next day. Two years later the same patient was reported in a Chicago newspaper as miraculously healed of yet another ailment. It was apparently another case of either the woman's extreme suggestibility or her shrewdness.

In a few months Locke and his allies moved the hospital three blocks south to a large, three-story brick house, until recently a well-known brothel. Its owner-proprietor had died. Locke officiated at her funeral, speaking "plainly and earnestly of the sinfulness of their lives" to parlorfuls of "abandoned women," some of them nearly hysterical with grief and worry. "It was a curious scene," he observed later.

The house's new owner rented it to Locke for his hospital. This new place was no better adapted for hospital use than the first one, but it was bigger. Now there was room for eighteen beds.

So far, Locke had not gone outside parish bounds for support. If he had, he wouldn't have gotten any, since "nearly everybody," including the bishop, Henry J. Whitehouse, "threw cold water on the project." The rector of St. James, then the city's leading parish, a friend of Locke, warned him against the project.

But Locke saw that it had to be more than a parish venture. Some well-known churchmen listened "good-naturedly" and agreed to be trustees when he laid his plan before them, though Locke was sure they thought he'd be better off attending to his parish.

One of them, Melville Fuller, a state legislator and later chief justice of the U.S. Supreme Court, shepherded a charter through the legislature. The trustees of the newly chartered hospital were the rector and a lay representative of each of the city's fourteen Episcopal parishes.

Bishop Whitehouse "began to thaw" on the question and in September of 1865 spoke "tolerably well" to the diocesan convention of what Locke called his "baby hospital." Others began to lend a hand, including "good women from all the parishes," who solicited donations in kind: "jams, jellies, fruits, flowers, cakes, and barrels of oysters."

But in 1868 Grace Church still bore most of the considerable expense. When things got tough, Locke would call the board together and threaten to close the place. The trustees "would hearten (him) up a little," and he would agree to go on.

Dr. John E. Owens became medical director in 1865. He held the position to 1911. The early staff included a number of Rush professors, including Dr. Hay, who reorganized the Chicago Health Department in 1867. Hay lectured on the brain and nervous diseases at Rush beginning in 1873. Later he organized Rush's department of neurology and was editor of *The Chicago Medical Journal.*

Dr. Moses Gunn, head of surgery at Rush, was a consulting surgeon at St. Luke's, as was Dr. William O. Heydock, a Chicago Medical College professor. Later staff members included Rush professors Dr. James H. Etheridge, a gynecologist, and Dr. Isaac N. Danforth, an early user of the microscope who in his later years was a kidney specialist.

The State Street house was almost comically inadequate. Autopsies were done on the dining room table. The staff found this unappetizing. Drugs were kept in the dining room. Ventilation was bad. A machine shop in the rear was dreadfully noisy. There was no good place to keep a corpse between expiration and burial.

The dining room doubled as a free dispensary from 1869. This was no problem. All it took was an "airing out," and it was ready to be a dining room again.

But "a great deal of earnest Christian work" was done at the State Street building, said Locke. Overseeing it all was the "matron" Sarah Miles. "How wise she was, how economical, how she hated whiskey and lies, and how far she could see through a stone wall!" Locke wrote in praise of this woman, the first superintendent of St. Luke's.

In 1869 an eye and ear department was added, with Dr. Samuel J. Jones in charge.

But Locke wanted out of the State Street place. The trustees were talking up a storm but no rain was falling, probably because six years after it was founded the hospital was operating at a grand annual surplus of $25. Finally John de Koven made his move.

De Koven, treasurer for the trustees and a warm friend of the young hospital, came to Locke with news that a big frame building was for sale on Indiana Avenue near 14th Street. The builder of a boarding house had gone broke and was looking for a buyer. De Koven urged Locke to buy the place. He put $2,000 of his own money where his advice was and promised fund-raising help besides. Others helped to raise more, including Mrs. John Tilden, who gave a concert, and Mrs. B. F. Hadduck, who held a fair. Millionaire lard manufacturer Nathaniel K. Fairbank, destined to be a major St. Luke's benefactor, gave $500.

The new place opened May 15, 1871, at 1426-30 South Indiana Avenue, with 25 beds bought with proceeds from a charity ball. All but a few were for charity patients, St. Luke's being for "the relief of respectable poor people," in Locke's words. As in its previous location, the hospital existed to "furnish a Christian home" where "the chaplain daily directs (patients') thoughts to God." The chaplaincy at this time was taken over by Reverend William Toll, Locke's assistant at Grace Church.

In the following October came the fire. Locke was at the Episcopal general convention in Baltimore. Worried sick, he hurried back by train but found his family safe and Grace Church and rectory unharmed, though furniture was piled on drays in case the fire came near. His assistant, Mr. Toll, had taken Locke's children and his sermons to the far South Side. The fire had stopped two blocks north of the church and three north of the hospital.

Locke thought the end had come for his "baby hospital," even if it had been spared, because he expected funds to dry up after the fire. But the fire was a mixed disaster. Two million dollars in relief money became available, and Mayor R. B. Mason assigned its management to the nine-year-old Chicago Relief & Aid Society—not to the city's aldermen, who were dying to get their hands on it. The society's members—including Grace parishioners N. K. Fairbank and Marshall Field —were citizens used to caring for the poor and sick.

This group turned to St. Luke's Hospital as "just the place for the sick and poor of the more respectable class." (For Locke respectability did not depend on solvency.) The society took over most of the hospital's operating expenses and gave it an additional $28,000, of which $16,000 was to be used to buy land.

St. Luke's in return was to hold 28 beds for use by the society when needed. (The society never used more than five at a time.) The $16,000 paid for a lot on State Street near 37th Street; the intention was to build a new hospital there. St. Luke's also received $4,000 from the Episcopal Church.

The Relief & Aid Society later matched a $4,000 hospital building fund which had survived the financial panic of 1873. In the same year, 1876, a free dispensary was opened. Locke fed eight to ten panhandlers a day at the hospital door with food left over from patients' meals until the trustees told him to stop, because it encouraged street begging.

"Of course, the wisdom of a Board of Trustees is unquestionable," observed the irrepressible priest. There were 12 trustees in all, a priest and two laymen from each side of the city. Locke called it "a curious arrangement, and very narrow." It was expected to increase church interest, "but it never did."

In 1878 E. K. Hubbard raised money for the long-awaited morgue, a nagging problem since the days on State Street. And George Chamberlain, a member of the St. Luke's medical board, did the same towards supplying hot water throughout the building. The first endowed bed, known as "the Churchman Cot for children," had been established with $3,000 raised by *The Churchman,* an Episcopal magazine in New York, which printed a "moving appeal" for small donations and listed contributors weekly.

Another early fund raiser was Mrs. Locke's sale of Angora cats at $25 each. It may indeed have been the first money raised for the hospital. Locke memorialized the effort with riddle-*cum*-doggerel: "How would you battle with sin and strife (precious wife)?" Answer: "With the simple Cat-echism." He called the women who helped his wife sell cats the "Cat club."

But major early contributions were in kind—fruit, vegetables, meat, linen supplies which flowed "without ceasing" into the St. Luke's storeroom. Not a cent was spent on hospital linen until the early 1890s. Locke's wife played a major role in keeping this philanthropic effort rolling, but others helped too.

Among them was Mrs. Joseph T. Ryerson, of the iron and steel family. Her "counsel and energy" were "invaluable," said Locke. Mrs. Ryerson's son Arthur was president of the St. Luke's trustees when she died in 1881, the same year Dr. M. O. Heydock, one of the first of the medical staff, died. Arthur Ryerson later succeeded Locke as president of the hospital.

Indeed, an era passed with Mrs. Ryerson's death. Gifts in kind slowed to a trickle by the mid-1890s, though the need was "ten times greater" because of the larger number of patients.

The institution was chartered a second time, in 1880, as St. Luke's Free Hospital. This was to take advantage of new legislation allowing not-for-profit organizations to hold assets of more than the $100,000 to which it was limited by the first charter. The name represented no change of policy. St. Luke's had been free to the needy from the beginning. In 1894 it was chartered a third time, and the hospital was again called simply St. Luke's.

Locke's "darling child," as he called St. Luke's, "took prodigious strides" in 1881. In that year N. K. Fairbank bought and gave to the hospital 100 feet of adjacent Indiana Avenue frontage, bringing this to 164 feet in all. Others at Fairbank's urging bought and donated 70 feet of Michigan Avenue frontage. Fairbank also helped raise money for a permanent structure.

The new building would be on the Indiana Avenue site, not farther south as had been planned. The advantages were its central location and proximity to lake and train stations. The trains' noise annoyed almost no patients but instead became "an unfailing source of entertainment" to the many railway employees who were patients at St. Luke's, Locke claimed.

Indeed, the Illinois Central Railroad endowed a bed and kept it occupied for over ten years with a series of injured employees. The hospital took care of IC accident victims, and the railroad responded generously, "paying well" for patients not covered by the endowed bed and otherwise showing the hospital "many favors."

When the cornerstone of the first "real hospital" was laid on All Saints Day, 1882, $57,000 was already subscribed, of which $25,000 was the gift of Dr. Tolman Wheeler. The rest had been solicited by Fairbank, much if not most of it from fellow Grace parishioners and civic leaders—meatpacker Philip D. Armour, retailer Marshall Field, wholesale grocer John W. Doane, and utilities investor Columbus R. Cummings. Mrs. Marshall Field raised $2,610 by holding a benefit concert at her home.

Dr. Wheeler helped St. Luke's in other ways and willed it a substantial piece of property. But shortly before he died in 1889, he sold the piece in question, having been "poisoned against" St. Luke's in his final days. "The hospital had a friendly visit with the heirs about this business, but lost the case," noted Locke.

Another potential benefactor, Thomas Lowther, coupled "crankiness" with his generosity, as in specifying that no married priest could live in the cathedral parish house for which he donated the lot, "a thing which . . . much hampered the bishop in his management of the cathedral." Lowther, a prominent promoter of a public library for the city, once offered Locke "a fine site" for St. Luke's, but Locke declined because of conditions he attached which Locke left unspecified.

A benefactor whom Locke called "peculiar" was George Armour, a Grace church member who built what in effect was a competitor church at 20th and State streets which eventually collapsed for lack of interest, including Armour's. Armour's eccentricity took a nice turn at the 1882 cornerstone ceremony, however, when he laid a $5,000 donation on the cornerstone.

St. Luke's moved into the new building January 29, 1885, $25,000 in debt. But Locke appealed in the press for funds to cover it and in a week had thousands more in hand. The new building forced St. Luke's to make changes, the first of which was to develop a nursing department. Four nurses—two men and two women—had handled everything in the old place, under Sarah Miles' guidance. But now there were wards and more complicated work to be done. The solution was to form a nurse-training program much like the Illinois Training School for Nurses. Thus was begun the St. Luke's training school for nurses in 1885, the 35th nurses' school in the U.S., organized on the Florence Nightingale model—that is, run by nurses (mostly women), rather than by doctors (mostly men).

Early candidates for the new school had to be high school graduates (though no proof was required for this) and had to be between 21 and 31 years old and of good family background and "upbringing." It was a period when nursing was coming into its own as work considered suitable for young women of "respectable" background.

Twelve of the first 29 students were graduates of Dearborn Seminary, a girls' private school. The rest were public school graduates. One of the early candidates came from Scotland, recommended by a galaxy of acquaintances that included the archbishop of Canterbury, a dozen nobles, several physicians, a veterinarian and the village blacksmith. Students came as individuals when openings occurred, as was typical of nursing schools of the day, not as groups or classes. The first six graduated in 1887, nine more in 1888.

The school's superintendent from 1888 to 1893 was Miss Catherine L. Lett. She died in office, mourned as "a devout daughter of the church" who left her life work "in the hearts and lives of others." Among other things, she set up a pay scale for graduate nurses of three dollars a day or $20 a week for general and surgical nursing, $25 a week for contagious disease work.

Life for the students was religious and disciplined. In fact, the acting chaplain, the Rev. George Todd, wanted to make of them a full fledged religious society, but Locke couldn't see it. They prayed before meals and sang in choir, even those connected to no church. None of these ever objected but were "thankful for the privilege," said Locke. A student was expelled for staying overnight in Waukegan without permission. Lett scolded another for going to hear a sermon by a dissenting clergyman.

A lighter side prevailed as well. When student and other nurses felt the need, they unburdened themselves to Mr. "Canary," as they called the owner of Carnegie's drug store, at 16th Street and Indiana Avenue. The English-born Maria, matron in charge of the nurses' residence, warned them that "ladies don't whistle." The now retired Sarah Miles in her wheelchair, Old John the baker and Ike the newsboy were other fixtures of hospital life.

In 1889, nurse alumnae formed the Blue Cross Society, to care for sick nurses and to strive for higher nursing standards and mutual encouragement. A room was set aside for sick nurses called the Blue Room. The blue cross, the society's emblem, was to be worn on the left arm "as a badge and token of service to the sick and suffering."

In 1896 this blue cross became part of the uniform, 38 years before a blue cross was first used by an office of the hospital insurance association of that name and 43 years before it was copyrighted by the American Hospital Association.

The uniform for street wear included a long gray cloak, little gray stringless bonnet edged with black velvet, and veil. The bonnet gave "a becoming look" and was said to "soften the face." It was worn until 1912.

The working uniform included an apron and an organdy hat that couldn't be flattened once it was assembled for wearing. The hat was carried in a hatbox to and from one's assignment, which was usually in a private home. (Nurses at Presbyterian Hospital, on the other hand, wore washable hats that could be carried flat.)

In 1939 white shoes and stockings were prescribed for St. Luke's nurses. The uniform came to mean much for students and alumnae. A St. Luke's graduate of the 1940s pleaded, "Don't let anyone change our caps—ever!" The plea was to take meaning during the sometimes difficult merger in the 1950s of the Presbyterian and St. Luke's schools of nursing.

The head of the St. Luke's medical staff, Dr. John E. Owens, took great pride in the new nursing school. The tall, bearded Owens made his late afternoon rounds with a red carnation in the buttonhole of his white coat and a friendly word for everyone. He became a much appreciated source of encouragement to nurses.

Housing the student nurses was a problem. Trustee Byron L. Smith, president of the Northern Trust Company, built a two-story addition on the West Pavilion (facing Michigan Avenue) for $13,000.

St. Luke's meanwhile was demonstrating a "quality of mercy not strained" to people of "all sects and nationalities," according to Rush Medical College Professor J. Adams Allen, a member of the St. Luke's consulting board, in remarks at the hospital's annual meeting.

This consulting board was dispensed with in 1887, notwithstanding Allen's kind remarks. Indeed, the whole medical board was reorganized, including the obstetrical and gynecological department, which was divided into two separate entities. Also that year, Dr. Moses Gunn died. He'd been senior attending surgeon, a Grace Church parishioner and a good friend of Locke, in addition to being for years the chairman of surgery at Rush.

The year also was marked by "large donations in kind," including "no small quantity of beer" from the Seipp Brewing Company and all the ice the hospital needed from the J. P. Smith Ice Company. In addition, Mrs. John Tilden solicited for the hospital "a very large amount of groceries."

But unspecified "petty squabbles" among members of the new medical board drove Locke "nearly frantic" in 1888. He "devoutly wished" to get a whole new medical staff at the time, as unwise as he knew that would be. Difficulties were ironed out, however; and "peace and harmony" reigned thenceforward.

To make matters worse, some "unknown person in our midst" was passing "garbled and childish information" to the press about internal matters, Locke wrote. He claimed he was stopped on the street in the midst of this and asked if St. Luke's burned babies in its furnace. "Yes we do, Madam," he said. "We find them cheaper than coal." The woman remained staring after Locke as he strode away.

Also in 1888 the State Street property (the former brothel)

was sold and the $25,000 proceeds were deposited in the endowment fund. The property would have been sold earlier for much less if N. K. Fairbank hadn't persuaded them to hold on to it. In the same year, an addition was begun in honor of the late Samuel Johnston, a landowner and traction executive who had left the hospital $55,000. This was finished in 1890, and a "noble pile" it was in Locke's estimation, "built with great economy." Its top story, he noted, was "beautifully fitted for pay patients," who, it should be added, had to be paying more than their share for St. Luke's to afford giving so much free care.

The addition doubled capacity, raising it to 152 beds, which in turn called for an increase in nurses. Housing them was again a challenge. The solution was to raise the training school department roof and add a floor. Mrs. E. H. Stickney footed this expense. Later, she willed St. Luke's its biggest gift so far, a $75,000 bequest which the hospital received in 1897. This went to build the Stickney House for nurses in 1898.

In fiscal 1889 the hospital cared for 1,050 patients, 611 of whom paid nothing. This total was well over the previous year's 817 and many times the 124 cared for in fiscal 1865, the first year. But there were still waiting lists; and people complained when they couldn't get in, exhibiting an "unreasonableness" which "much tried" Locke and the staff. It was a wonderful year nonetheless. Railroad car magnate George M. Pullman and his daughter contributed to the children's ward and helped make it "the most beautiful and complete home for sick children in this country." In the hospital as a whole, Locke reported, "harmony reigned in every department."

The operating deficit rose to $30,000, however. A partial solution was to use invested endowment funds to build an apartment building on Michigan Avenue in back of the hospital, in the hope of earning a greater return. The new building was called "The Clinton" in honor of Locke. For a year or so, it gave a better return, perhaps because of increased demand for housing during the world's fair. In 1899 it was rebuilt after a fire and renamed "The Saranac," possibly after the vacation and health resort in the Adirondacks.

Meanwhile, in fiscal 1892, 59 percent of St. Luke's efforts

went for charity patients and much of the rest was only "part pay." On the poorest patients as on the rich, the medical staff "lavished every attention" at a per-patient per year cost of $47.66, which did not reflect the "great quantities" of linen and bedding supplied by members of Grace and another Episcopal church, Trinity.

Fund raising by individuals remained a major advantage. Helen K. Fairbank, wife of Nathaniel, worked especially hard soliciting funds for endowed beds, sometimes in amounts as low as $5 and $10. At her death a ward was named in her honor.

The 1893 world's fair gave St. Luke's a chance to shine. The hospital was full "almost constantly," Locke reported, and nurse Grace Critchell Tracy walked 25 miles a night covering the wards. She knew this thanks to a pedometer she wore to track her perambulations.

At the fairgrounds several miles to the south, 12,000 lived. Dr. Owens ran an emergency hospital there for fairgoers and workers. Three of its four nurses were from St. Luke's.

Another emergency that engaged the St. Luke's staff was the 1903 Iroquois theatre fire which killed 571 and loaded St. Luke's morgue beyond capacity. People lined up to identify their dead. St. Luke's was also called on after the capsizing of the excursion steamer Eastland at its docking place in the Chicago River in 1915, when 812 drowned.

Two turn-of-the-century St. Luke's physicians of note were Dr. Henry Baird Favill, of Rush, and Dr. Robert B. Preble. Favill could stand in a ward and "smell measles" among the patients, the story goes. "Let me see that case of bronchitis you admitted this morning," he once asked, and discovered a measles rash.

Favill, a Rush alumnus and longtime Rush faculty member, succeeded Owens as president of the St. Luke's medical staff. He was the son of a physician of English ancestry but a descendent on his mother's side of an Ottawa Indian chief and proud of it. When his wife was inducted into the Colonial Dames, he was asked if he qualified for the Society of Mayflower Descendents. "No," he answered, "my people were on the reception committee.''

Preble, an internist who later joined Herrick, Billings and others in forming the Society of Internal Medicine in Chicago, was also a canny diagnostician. Faced on one occasion with a presumed case of gastric hemorrhage, he expressed immediate doubt, lifted the sheet and discovered what he suspected, the dilated veins that showed cirrhosis of the liver.

Surgery in the late 19th century was sometimes performed in people's homes. Not always, however. St. Luke's may have been the scene of an historic first in 1894, when Daniel Hale Williams, a black surgeon on the St. Luke's staff, is said to have performed heart surgery. Some question this, saying the first such operation was performed in St. Louis.

The medical historian Thomas N. Bonner doesn't even mention it in relation to Williams, whom he does credit with a similar first, not at St. Luke's but at Chicago's Provident Hospital, which Williams helped to found. This operation, an emptying and suturing of the pericardial sac in the chest of a stabbing victim in 1893, was noteworthy in any event, heart surgery or not and the first of its kind or not.

St. Luke's was the scene in 1898 of what may have been the first Caesarean section in the Midwest. Nurses watched it from ''the long windows'' of what in 1946 was known as the ''old building,'' shrieking in subdued fashion when the baby appeared. The director of the nurses' school was ''victorianly shocked'' at her nurses witnessing the event, says Marie Merrill in her history of the nursing school. The baby's parents wrote the trustees to thank them, noting, ''Being poor, we have nothing to give you, but will give small things whenever we can afford to.''

Money problems abounded. Like the reputedly wealthy English hospitals, St. Luke's had to operate regularly at a deficit, trusting donations to keep it in what was essentially a catch-up ball game. One problem was lack of sufficient endowment.

Another was how to afford the latest in medical equipment—special splints or braces for patients suffering from hunchback, curvature of the spine, club feet and the like. Most were able to pay little or nothing toward the cost of such apparatus. The problem presaged huge expenditures of a coming age, when new equipment was to cost far more than splint and braces.

A related problem was what to do about nonpaying patients, who usually stayed longer than paying ones because the hospital was more comfortable than anywhere else they had to go. Locke does not say how he solved this problem.

In 1885 Locke resigned as president of St. Luke's and was succeeded by Arthur Ryerson. The end of an era came with the end of Locke's involvement. As its first president and chaplain, he was a beloved figure and a genuine human being. In 1895 his vocal organs gave way, and he had to call a halt to his pastoral work. At first he couldn't preach, then he couldn't talk at all. An "awful silence" ensued, Bishop McLaren wrote. "The charm of life vanished," and he "longed for the death he did not fear."

Locke took to playing cribbage at the hospital, where he went apparently as much for companionship as anything else. Locke died in 1904 on the Mississippi gulf coast, where he and his wife were vacationing. He was 74 years old, the oldest priest in the diocese. Adele Locke, his helpmate in pastoral labors, spent her final years at the Grace Church rectory on Indiana Avenue. She died in 1919 at 79.

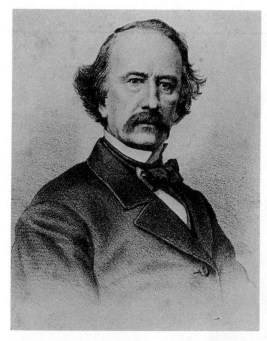

Daniel Brainard, M.D., 1812–1866.

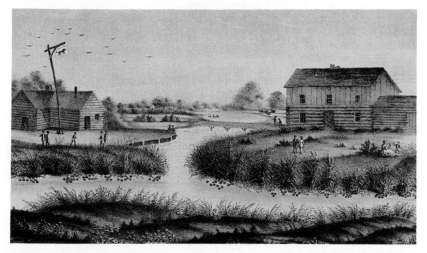

"Wolf's Point in 1833."
(Photo courtesy Chicago Historical Society)

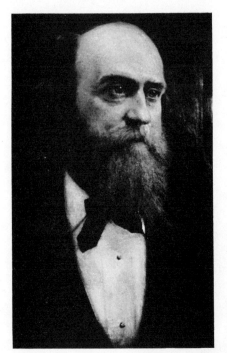

James Van Zandt Blaney,
M.D., 1820–1874.

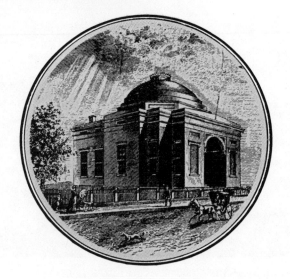

Rush Medical College, 1844.

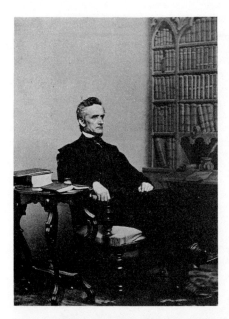

Nathan Smith Davis, M.D.,
1817–1904. *(Photo courtesy of
Chicago Historical Society)*

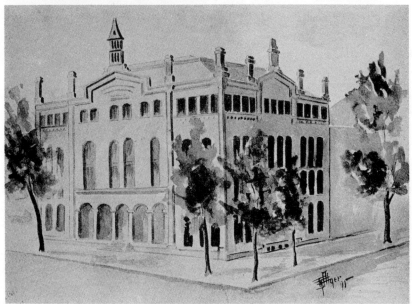

Rush Medical College building of 1867.
(Photo courtesy of Chicago Historical Society)

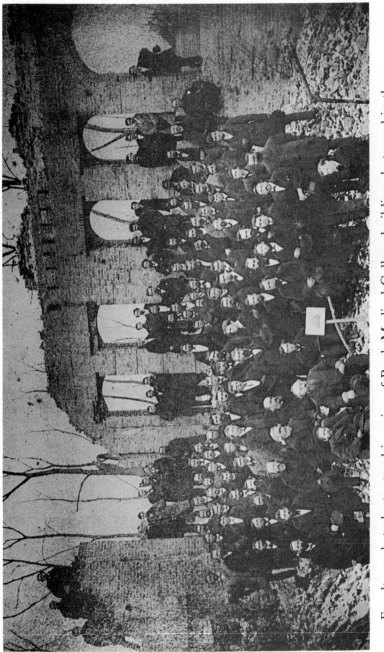

Faculty and students stand in ruins of Rush Medical College building destroyed in the Chicago Fire of 1871.

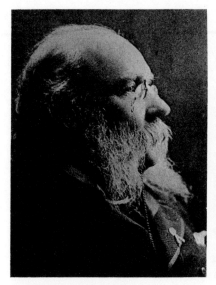

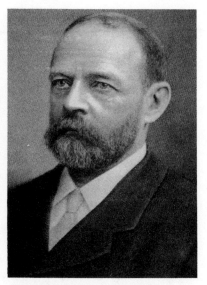

Moses Gunn, M.D.,
1822–1887: "A surgeon must
have the eye of a hawk, the
heart of a lion, the hand of a
woman."

Christian Fenger, M.D.,
1840–1902.

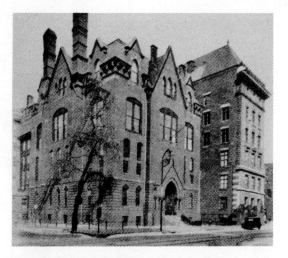

Rush Medical College, 1875 building, and
Senn Building (right), added in 1902.

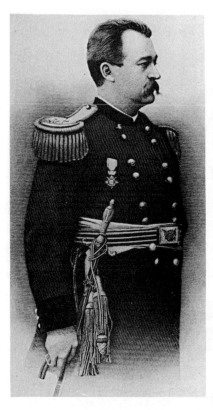

Nicholas Senn, M.D.,
1844–1908.

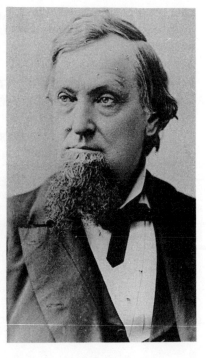

Joseph P. Ross, M.D.,
1828–1890.

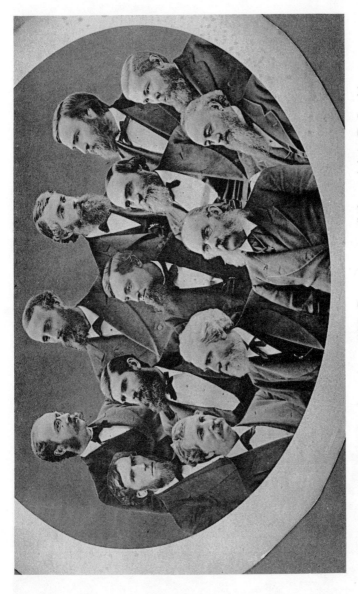

Rush Medical College faculty, circa 1875. Bottom row: (left to right), DeLaskie Miller, J. W. Freer, Moses Gunn, J. A. Allen. Second row: E. L. Holmes, R. L. Rea, Joseph P. Ross, J. V. Z. Blaney, Walter Hay. Third row: J. H. Etheridge, N. Bridge, H. M. Lyman, C. T. Parkes.

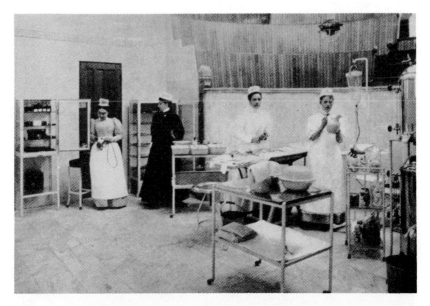

Corwith Memorial Operating Room of Presbyterian Hospital, 1895.

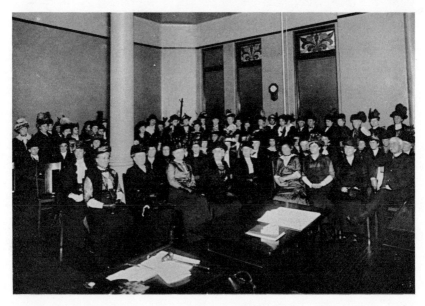

Presbyterian Hospital Woman's Auxiliary, circa. 1910.

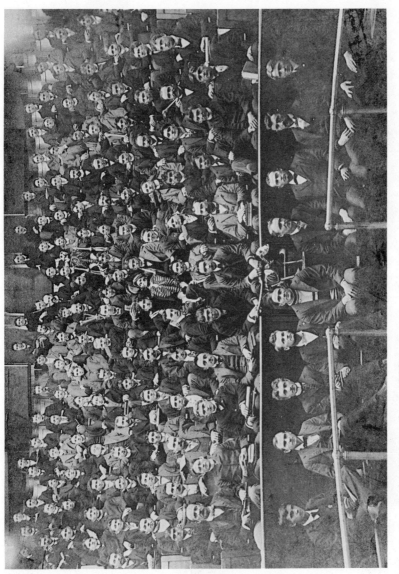

Rush medical students, late 1890s.

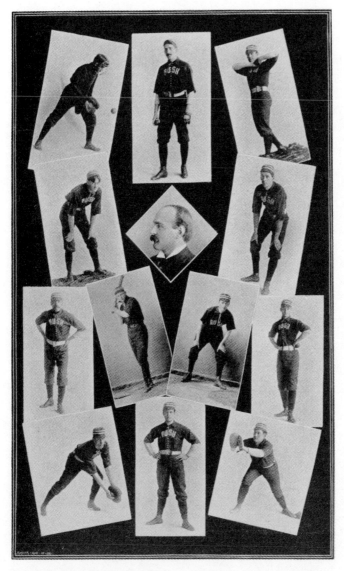

Rush baseball team, 1894.

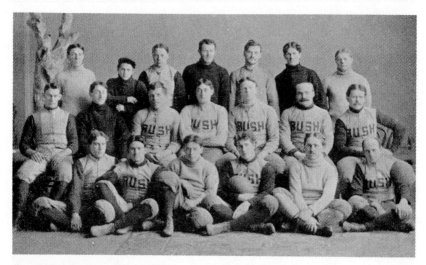

Rush football team, 1894.

DATE	OPPONENTS	RUSH		OPPONENTS
Sept. 22.	WEST DIVISION HIGH SCHOOL, - - -	42	to	0
Sept. 29.	PRAIRIE CLUB, Oak Park, Ill., - - - -	12	to	0
Oct. 13.	UNIVERSITY OF CHICAGO, - - - -	6	to	16
Oct. 20.	CHICAGO ATHLETIC ASSOCIATION, - - -	6	to	12
Oct. 27.	BELOIT COLLEGE, at Beloit, Wis., - -	12	to	22
Nov. 3.	LAKE FOREST UNIVERSITY, - - - -	34	to	6
Nov. 22.	NOTRE DAME UNIVERSITY, at South Bend, Ind.,	6	to	6
Nov. 25.	IOWA COLLEGE, at Grinnell, Iowa, - - -	6	to	28
Nov. 29.	MONMOUTH COLLEGE, at Monmouth, Ill., -	18	to	6

The 1894 football season.

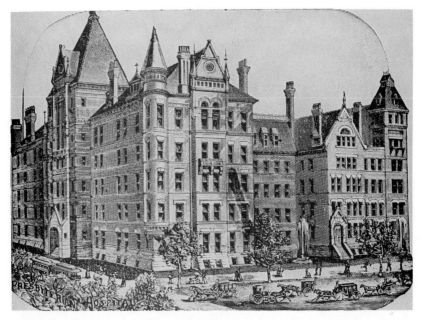

Jones Building of Presbyterian Hospital with Ross-Hamill Wing at right, late 1880s.

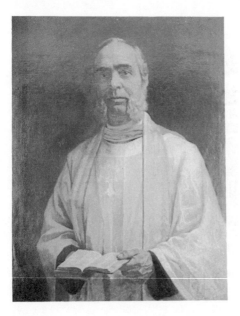

The Reverend James De Witt Clinton Locke, 1829–1904, pastor of Grace Episcopal Church and founder of St. Luke's Hospital.

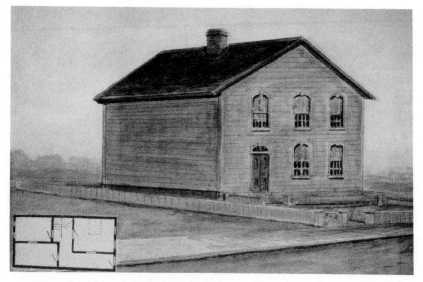

The first St. Luke's Hospital, 1864.
(Photo courtesy of Chicago Historical Society)

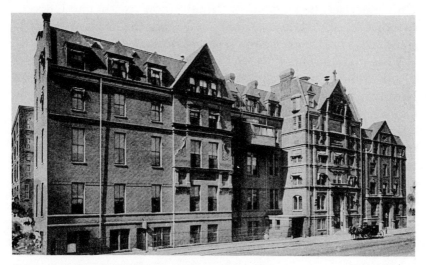

St. Luke's Hospital old main building, 1882.

A Marriage Made In Heaven: Rush & The University Of Chicago 1898-1924

The final split of Rush Medical College from Lake Forest University set the stage for a "final union" with The University of Chicago. It was a marriage made in heaven by most standards, but nevertheless destined to end on the rocks.

The matchmakers were Doctors E. Fletcher Ingals and Frank Billings on the Rush side (though Billings was then at Northwestern University Medical School) and University of Chicago President William Rainey Harper on the other.

Ingals was a Rush teacher (since 1871), trustee and its controller. He realized the Lake Forest connection was worth little to either party, partly because Lake Forest would never attract endowment funds sufficient to help Rush achieve its potential. In the dealings with Harper, Ingals played a crucial role.

At one point he alone among Rush trustees voted for affiliation. Deputed to inform Harper of the deal-killing vote, he persuaded the others to wait a while. It was that close to not happening.

Billings, a distinguished medical practitioner and researcher with an itch to promote medical education, was winning a reputation for getting things done. As secretary of the faculty at Northwestern, he had helped build Wesley Hospital and a new classroom structure. He was later to resign over what he considered Northwestern trustees' failure to support the medical school adequately.

Ingals saw possibilities in the new university and went to work on Harper immediately with his Rush affiliation idea. Billings joined him in the effort in a year or two, so that by 1893 or 1894, they both were after Harper. It took a few years more, but by December of 1897, Harper liked the idea, under four nonnegotiable conditions:

1. The Rush trustees would resign in favor of new ones with "no pecuniary interest" in Rush's earnings, named by the University trustees. Gone were the days when Rush was "what would now be termed a proprietary medical school," to use Rush alumni president Dr. H. Gideon Wells' 1922 expression. Proprietors or not, Wells hastened to add, they were dedicated, idealistic men.

2. Rush entrance requirements would be raised to two years of college by 1902. This drastically cut the number of eligible students, since only 10 or 12% of high-school graduates entered college at the time. Later enrollment dropped accordingly.

3. Rush would retire its debt.

4. The Rush faculty would resign and await reappointment by the university.

A Rush man asked how they knew Harper would reappoint Rush men. They didn't, a colleague replied. But either Harper knew what he was doing or didn't. If he didn't, they shouldn't affiliate. If he did, they shouldn't tie his hands.

The affiliation was neither a union of the two schools nor a commitment to one, Harper emphasized. It left both parties' options open. But University of Chicago founder John D. Rockefeller was still not pleased. He and his advisor Frederick T. Gates felt the university lowered itself by the union partly because Rush trained practitioners, not researchers.

Harper, on the other hand, saw that Rush and University of

Chicago goals might be joined to make something new and grand in U.S. medical history. He saw Rush as something he could mold into the medical school with everything: it would educate both scientifically trained practitioners and researchers.

Harper went at the molding process with vigor, beginning with an 18-point agreement he produced for Rush signatures, a document that included the four basic conditions and added other details:

The university would examine and approve applicants at Rush's expense. It would furnish "at cost" teachers, books and supplies and would lend books and apparatus "at net cost of transit and handling." Rush would do nothing academic without university approval, including hiring and firing faculty. Rush would raise student requirements "as rapidly as the university may require."

On top of all this, Harper put it in writing (and Rush gladly signed) that (a) nothing in the above implied encouragement that Rush would ever become the university's medical school, and (b) the university intended to establish such a school of its own as soon as money was available.

The whole deal was, on its face, no bargain for Rush. But if the Rush people were bargain-hunting, they wouldn't have dealt with Harper, whom they revered as a medical-education Moses who would lead them to glory. On January 5, 1898, the seven Rush trustees—Professors Holmes, Lyman, Etheridge, Ingals, Hyde, Haines and Bridge—resigned, and eight university trustees, including food-wholesaler A. A. Sprague, were appointed in their places.

The faculty retired the debt as stipulated—$73,000 incurred six years earlier to build the Rush laboratory building. Dr. Nicholas Senn, the surgeon, and Ingals each came up with $25,000, and others supplied the rest.

In June the affiliation became official, and the Rush faculty asked Harper to be president. He declined the title but assumed the responsibility, presiding at faculty meetings and appointing committees. He also persuaded the faculty to democratize itself by giving the vote, previously the preserve of an 11-man executive committee, to all above assistant professor. He argued that this would balance conservative and progressive influence. Faculty meetings weren't for voting anyhow, he explained, but for mutual education.

Education was necessary, since radical changes were in store. Whatever the 1894 Rush yearbook had said in favor of practical experience, lectures were still the norm. Students sat on amphitheatre benches eight or nine hours a day, listening or watching. The course was rigid and inflexible and the same for all. The university was trying other methods, and so would Rush.

Rush, which operated eight months a year, became a year-round school. The earliest Rush students had gone only four months a year. Later an optional spring session had been added. Now the year was divided into quarters, and students could attend all four quarters and still have seven weeks' vacation. Faculty could teach two or three four-quarter years and then take a year or 18 months off for study. The student needed 12 quarters to graduate but had to take 45 months to do it, because of state requirements.

Furthermore, the curriculum was reorganized to reflect what students could do, rather than what teachers thought necessary to cover the subject. Thus eight or nine hours a day for five or five and a half days the first two years and six days the second two years would be realistic goals. Another change, a medical school first, was the institution of electives. The purpose was pedagogical. Choosing courses was an event in itself. On at least one occasion, students stood in line from a little after midnight to be sure they got the course of their choice.

Another change was the admission of women, again to conform to University of Chicago practice. The first, in 1901, were received with no more "altered demeanor" among male students "than if an equal number of men had been added to the student body," according to Dean of Students John Milton Dodson. By 1917, 68 women had graduated.

Another momentous change occurred in 1901, one for which Ingals and Billings argued at length: Rush freshmen and sophomores moved to the South Side university campus for basic science classes—the first two years of the curriculum.

Rush Medical College on the West Side at this point became a two-year school, educating only third- and fourth-year medical students in their clinical or "clerkship" studies. Incoming Rush freshman took classes on the South Side and enrolled as students of both Rush and the university.

The move not only pleased the Rush leadership but also fitted into Harper's plans for a medical school whose first two years were "almost entirely courses in pure science." Rush students had to be sold, however. Horse-drawn coaches were hired one day in May, and the freshmen were driven out south to view their new surroundings, eat lunch and hear from Harper and others the advantages of a University of Chicago education.

Harper was as persuasive with them as he had been with the faculty, and all but a few continued their studies on the Midway the following September as students in the university's Ogden Graduate School of Science. Third- and fourth-year students continued on the West Side, where Billings became dean of faculty and Dr. John Milton Dodson became dean of students.

Other medical schools followed suit and offered pure science in the first two years. Third- and fourth-year students from many of these schools transferred to Rush for clinical studies. In fact, during the next 15 years, up to half the Rush enrollment hailed from elsewhere than The University of Chicago and never less than 20 percent.

A year after Ingals and Billings argued successfully for the move to the university campus for basic science, they went for even closer "organic union" with the university. This organic union would make Rush an integral part of the university, rather than a mere affiliate or working partner. Harper favored it, notwithstanding his proviso four years before, when he cautioned Rush not to get its hopes up. On the contrary, by 1903 he was convinced the university's medical school future lay with Rush.

What he wanted was something he could call the "Rush School of Medicine of The University of Chicago." So apt a partner had Rush already proven and such was its rich history, that the name alone was worth a million dollars, he said. Full of enthusiasm, he persuaded the university trustees and went off to New York to persuade the founder, Rockefeller.

He did so, but not completely. In any event, in order to be finally united with the university, Rush had to raise a million to qualify for the needed $5 million from the man who so far had made everything possible. Billings went to work with his usual energy, and the million was raised almost immediately.

But more than a third of it was a donation in kind, namely the McCormick Institute for Infectious Diseases, which Billings persuaded the Harold Fowler McCormicks to give to Rush. It wasn't unfettered cash with which to endow research, which is what Rockefeller had in mind.

No deal, said the philanthropist, and Harper was ready to tear his hair out. "I shall resign," he threatened, pacing back and forth in front of his deans at the Chicago Club. Indeed, he was looking at a tempting offer from the St. Louis world's fair to be director of its scientific and educational section. He would have taken it, but Rockefeller and the trustees talked him out of it.

His frustration lay in seeing a medical school so near and yet so far. Everything was ready for his grand plan:

• A five-pavilion, 250-bed research hospital on the South Side that would take patients of its choice from its outpatient department and other hospitals, based on the disease to be studied.

• The Rush complex on the West Side for undergraduate clinical work.

• A postgraduate school on the Near North Side. Chicago Policlinic School, at Chicago Avenue and LaSalle Street, was ready to become Rush's postgraduate school and bring its Henrotin Hospital as part of the bargain.

Research would be pursued at all three of these centers, and the staffs of each would use facilities of the others.

None of it happened in 1904. Harper entered Presbyterian Hospital early in the year for an appendectomy. Cancer was suspected but not found. A year later, exploratory surgery found it. A year after that, in February of 1906, he was dead. So was his dream of organic union—the absorption or integration of Rush—at least in its particulars and at least for another 20 years.

Meanwhile, as Rush's admission standards rose, its enrollment declined. Only 65 freshmen entered in 1905—a steep drop from 250 a few years earlier. It could have been worse. Rush raised its standards over a five-year period. Some schools raised theirs all at once and sank to as few as six freshmen, not even a baseball team.

Rush had enough for several baseball teams but still not enough to pay the bills. Many of the faculty were asked to forego their small stipends. Those who had pledged to give toward the million required by Rockefeller were asked to give to help meet current expenses. As dean of faculty, Billings solicited from potential donors. As controller, Ingals managed astutely. In a few years, the students began to return, even with the higher standards limiting the pool. By 1910 Rush enrollment topped 360, up from 253 in 1905, and the crisis had passed.

The question remained abut organic union. Harper's successor, Harry Pratt Judson, assured Billings, Dodson, and Ingals of his interest but said the matter should remain on hold. He took up where Harper had left off as a Rush trustee and de facto president but not as its champion in the halls of the mighty. Four years later, even the mighty took his leave. Rockefeller pulled out in 1910, promising the university a final $10 million over the next 10 years, including $1.5 million for a chapel.

Rush's big three—Billings, Dodson and Ingals—again approached the university, this time with the American Medical Association stalwart and Rush professor, Dr. Arthur Dean Bevan, at their side. Billings put it to Martin Ryerson, president of the university trustees: would they rather Rush went its own way while the university formed its medical school? Ryerson's answer was that they would not. They wanted Rush to remain in affiliation, just as it was, until something stronger might develop.

A strain was developing nonetheless. Rush had no money to speak of. Billings was again given the task of raising some. But no big plans were there to inspire giving, and Rush's future was unclear.

To complicate matters further, other institutions were looking around, including the University of Illinois, which had taken over the College of Physicians and Surgeons in 1913. Illinois proposed organic union with Rush, but with the smell about it of annexation. Rush would surrender its charter, disband its trustees and give up its name. Furthermore, while the (tax) money was there, legislators controlled it year by year, and Rush shied away from that dependency. The Rush faculty said no to Illinois in April of 1914. Northwestern University Medical School also approached Rush with a view to union. This didn't happen either.

Then in the summer of 1916, Billings, ever the planner and promoter, presented Rockefeller interests with three options for the university's medical education: move it all to the South Side, move it all to the West Side, or move only Rush's undergraduate clinical education south and make Rush a postgraduate medical school.

The Rockefeller organization, in the person of medical education expert Abraham Flexner, liked the third option, which was a variation of Harper's plan for research south, undergraduate education west and postgraduate education north.

Money again was the problem, but this time it was solved in rapid fashion. Billings raised in record time (a matter of months) the $3.3 million required by the Rockefeller Foundation and the General Education Board, each of which promised $1 million. His family gave $1 million, including $400,000 from his cousin Cornelius K. G. Billings, former president of People's Gas, and $100,000 from himself. He solicited the rest almost entirely from Rosenwald, Ryerson, Armour, Swift and other philanthropic sources.

Banker Frederick H. Rawson and his wife gave $300,000 for a laboratory on the West Side, where Presbyterian Hospital and Rush were to form a European-style "university college" (postgraduate school of medicine) for M.D. practitioners.

Albert Merritt Billings Hospital on the South Side—named after an uncle of Frank, also a former head of People's Gas—was to be fully endowed and run on a "strictly scientific basis," without "any element of commercial medical practice," said university president Judson. It was to be controlled by staff, who would have no duties but to teach and do research and research-related clinical work.

The Rockefeller grant and accompanying plans made page one around the country. *The Chicago Tribune* called the idea "one of the most important events in the history of Chicago." The *Boston Transcript* said the grant gave the university its opportunity to form the nation's premier medical school. *The Nation* said the "new move at Chicago" would greatly help U.S. medical education meet the best European standards.

Congratulations were premature, however. It was wartime, and the grand plans had to be delayed. Not until several years after the war were they realized, in 1924. According to agreement Rush kept its name, and construction was begun on the new building on which were carved the words "Rawson Laboratory, Rush Postgraduate School of Medicine. A.D. 1924. The University of Chicago." On the South Side, Billings Hospital was begun.

The Rawson building held offices, library, classrooms and laboratories, including the fifth-floor pathology labs named after Dr. Norman Bridge, who with his wife had given $100,000 for their construction. In the basement was occupational therapy and on the second floor the Central Free Dispensary—moved there from Senn Hall, the 1902 five-story laboratory building next to it, named after the famous surgeon, Dr. Nicholas Senn, who gave $50,000 to help build it.

The affiliated institutions which gave Rush its strong clinical-education base were adjacent or nearby: the 440-bed Presbyterian Hospital, the McCormick Institute for Infectious

Diseases, the Home for Destitute Crippled Children. County Hospital was on the opposite corner.

On the South Side, Doctors Franklin McLean and Dean Lewis set to work organizing the undergraduate clinical program meant some day to replace Rush's clinical program.

In May of 1924, Rush and the university signed the agreement which joined them in marriage-like union. On June 7, the day after the Rush graduation, the Rush faculty and students became University of Chicago faculty and students.

In August the old Rush building was torn down to make way for Rawson. A cornerstone removal ceremony on August 28 was presided over by A. E. Wood, grand master of the lodge which had performed the cornerstone-laying ceremony not quite 50 years earlier.

Rush & The University of Chicago Go Their Separate Ways 1924-1941

Their marriage consummated in 1924, Rush Medical College and The University of Chicago upgraded requirements. A bachelor's degree was made compulsory. (Ten years earlier, Rush had been the first U.S. medical college to enforce the intern year requirement.) The new postgraduate school of medicine (for M.D. practitioners) was begun as the presumed justification of Rush as a university appendage. The M.D. undergraduate program was to be moved south as soon as possible.

On the West Side, Dr. Ernest E. Irons was the new dean. Here Rush continued to offer the third and fourth (clinical-education) years leading to the M.D. degree. These were the years of learning applied medicine, after years one and two spent on basic science courses on the South Side. Most clinical-education students, or "clerks" as they were called, came to Rush from the university's South Side campus. But quite a few came after taking basic science courses at some other medical school.

The mid-1920s to early 1930s were a sort of extended

76

honeymoon period for Rush and the university. The university contributed to Rush's new postgraduate school, and Rush alumni pledged $250,000 as their share of $3 million being raised by university alumni.

Identification was legally complete between the two institutions. It seems to have been morally complete as well. In addition to giving substantial help to university fund raising, Rush professors attended university functions such as the trustees' dinner for faculty at the South Shore Country Club and performed university duties such as serving on the university senate.

Rush's role in postgraduate medicine was to be "dominant," according to a university spokesman. The Rawson building which undergirded this role was dedicated in December of 1925, a five-story, all-steel structure connected by walkways to Senn Memorial on one side and Presbyterian Hospital on the other.

Rush's laboratory and classroom facilities put even Northwestern to shame, not to mention its principal claim to medical educational excellence—its proximity and working relationship with Presbyterian Hospital and the Central Free Dispensary.

The postgraduate program proceeded sluggishly, however. The offerings were generous: one to three years in otolaryngology, dermatology, ophthalmology or radiology. But only 20 enrolled in its first year. Dean Irons suggested a harder sell. He reported optimistically that a "week of clinics" during Rush Homecoming Week in June of 1926 had been well attended.

Rush's undergraduate (clinical) program, on the other hand, became increasingly attractive. Of 141 M.D. recipients in 1926, only 78 had done their first two (basic science) years at The University of Chicago. The rest had transferred from other medical schools. The university was becoming for Rush one of many feeder schools offering basic science (preclinical) courses.

At the same time the university was well on its way to the goal of offering a full four-year undergraduate program (basic science and clinical) on the South Side. The 1924 plan to which Rush had agreed was essentially what the Rockefeller organization's Abraham Flexner had worked out in 1916 with Frank Billings. Undergraduate medical education was to be on the South Side campus, postgraduate on the West Side. According to agreement, Rush was providing undergraduate clinical study only until the university could do it on the South Side.

But the Rush faculty thought or hoped it wouldn't turn out that way. They looked instead for a continuance of the status quo, apparently ignoring signs to the contrary, such as the Billings Hospital development with its promise of taking over Rush's clinical education role.

Rush graduated 142 M.D.s in 1927, of whom 98 had done preclinical work on the South Side. Rush's clinical and laboratory capacities were at a peak, with the new Rawson building in use for a year or so and increased cooperation reported with Presbyterian. The Central Free Dispensary cared for over 107,000 patients.

The death knell was sounding nonetheless. On October 10, 1927, the university opened for business on the South Side a full-service, four-year medical school. Rush faculty who cherished hopes of continuing to give undergraduate education must have found that unsettling.

The university now had two medical schools, one on the South Side staffed mainly by "so-called 'full-time' men," as acting President Frederic Woodward called them, the other on the West Side staffed by part-timers.

This was an important distinction. These "full-time men" were new for Chicago. They represented a system promoted by the Rockefeller organization, which had gotten the idea from the John Hopkins School of Medicine in Baltimore. The idea was that medical school teachers were to be free of the distraction of patient work except as it contributed directly to research. This freedom from the requirements of patient care cost money, of course; these men were on salary and responsible only to the medical school. Thus they were "full-timers."

From its start the university's South Side medical school program of the 1920s was based on full-time or "whole-time" salaried faculty. In charge of it was Rush alumnus and

Rockefeller-group protégé Dr. Franklin C. McLean. The pattern here was of the professional teacher as opposed to the teacher who is primarily a practitioner. It made sense in view of the university's commitment to medical research. It did not make sense where money was a concern.

At Rush, on the West Side, for instance, the full-timer was nonexistent. Nor, apparently, did the Rush teacher feel distracted from teaching by his practice, which he clearly felt contributed to his teaching while it paid the bills. Thirty years later, the full-timer issue was to rise at Presbyterian Hospital, during its postwar revival period.

The new South Side clinical undergraduate program ran into trouble at first, apparently because of its research orientation. Students who came to learn medicine were apparently put off by the number of electives, for instance—one out of three courses. Only those of "exceptionally clear vision and research ability" were expected to like the new program, said Dean Basil C. H. Harvey.

Each student was encouraged to pursue his or her interests; such was the belief in the educational value of research. The emphasis was on nurturing habits, rather than on transmitting information required by state licensing boards. Not all saw the value of this approach, lamented Harvey, who expected the program to be "relatively unpopular" for a few years.

Rush's future was being discussed. The university trustees announced it was to remain one of the university's two medical schools. Acting President Woodward acknowledged "differences in organization, method and emphasis" and said he hoped experience would show the way to reconciling them. The two schools "should complement each other with valuable results," he said. The Rush faculty was free to take what comfort they might from this oracular comment.

They were also free to judge as they might the next major announcement from the university—the appointment, effective July 1, 1929, of the young dean of the Yale law school, Robert Maynard Hutchins, as its fifth president. Hutchins was installed in November. One of his early pronouncements was to acclaim Rush Medical College as "a jewel in the crown" of the university. The Rush faculty was to have time to meditate on this encomium and to wonder what the new president had in mind when he bestowed it.

On the South Side, McLean as professor of medicine and Dr. Dallas B. Phemister as his counterpart in surgery were encountering "enormous" difficulties in organizing departments from scratch. As we have seen, McLean had overall responsibility for the new school, which he was creating on the approved Johns Hopkins model with an entirely full-time staff. He had organized the Rockefeller-sponsored Peking Union Medical College along the same lines. An apparently selfless individual, he put the whole South Side operation together but apparently stepped on some toes in the process and had to resign his supervisory position in December of 1932.

McLean and Phemister were joined in 1927 by Dr. Emmett B. Bay, also from Rush, who headed a cardiology section in the department of medicine. The new program was competing with Rush for faculty. It began also to compete for students. Students now had their choice of finishing on the South Side or at Rush. At first, they all took Rush, which was the proven commodity and offered superb clinical-education opportunities. But as Billings Hospital and the other university "clinics" became established, more chose the South Side.

The presence of highly respected former Rush teachers added to the appeal of the South Side campus. Phemister in 1925 had set up the first "full-time" surgery department in the world, leaving a lucrative private practice to do so. Bay had become the first physician to practice on the university's campus. Researcher George F. Dick became chairman of medicine in 1933. Neurologist Richard B. Richter came in 1936. Department of medicine members Doctors Walter L. Palmer, C. Philip Miller, Louis Leiter and Russell M. Wilder were Rush-University of Chicago alumni who also joined the South Side school. Wilder chaired medicine from 1929 to 1931, before Dick took over. All in all, the situation had a distinctly Rush-University of Chicago flavor to it.

The university "clinics" (the term covered the hospitals as well as the Max Epstein clinic) reached a bed capacity of over

500 by the early thirties, with a 500-a-day outpatient capacity. To medicine and surgery had been added obstetrics-cum-gynecology, pediatrics, and orthopedics. Billings Hospital had 216 beds, Bobs Roberts Memorial Hospital for Children (now part of the Wyler's Children's Hospital) had 80, Chicago Lying-In had 140 and the McElwee and Hicks hospitals provided a 100-bed orthopedic unit—all on the university campus.

In addition to these, the affiliated Children's Memorial Hospital, in the North Side's Lincoln Park area, accounted for 250 beds. The formidable West Side clinical-education complex was not overshadowed by all this, but like the long-distance runner in a hard race, it was hearing footsteps.

Not that Rush was standing still. Frank Billings gave $100,000 for four fellowships in 1930. Nancy Adele McElwee, a prominent benefactress of the South Side program, gave $500,000 for a surgical pavilion. Both gifts were part of what Rush and Presbyterian Hospital were presenting as a "comprehensive plan" for their joint development.

But it was time for the Hutchins factor to assert itself. In June of 1931, the "boy wonder" president told Rush graduates, alumni and friends that the university still didn't know what to do with Rush. "We must have either one school or two on a different basis," he said. Costs prohibited development of two "first-class" institutions.

This was waving a distress signal in front of Frank Billings, who stood up and told the audience he could raise the money they needed. "I'm 77 years old now," said the old campaigner. "But if I live to the time when we campaign for funds . . . I'll do as big a job as [I did] in 1917, when I raised two and a half million."

About this time Billings went to Alfred T. Carton, Sr., president of the Presbyterian Hospital's board of managers, with tears in his eyes to ask Carton to move the hospital to the South Side. Billings saw this as the move that would preserve the Rush–University of Chicago connection, and he desperately wanted to see it happen. He never did, of course.

In a few years, rumors flying, Rush students met to protest their coming "affiliation" with the university, according to a news account. But affiliation was hardly the issue. Rush was already part of the university. The issue was whether remaining a part of it would require a closing down of Rush undergraduate medical education or even of Rush itself on the West Side. Dean Irons told the students nothing "immediate" was being considered. University Vice President Woodward told the press that merger had been discussed.

This merger discussion had included an offer to the senior attending staff of Presbyterian Hospital to come to the South Side campus. The university would give land on which Presbyterian could be built anew. But the Presbyterian's bylaws required it to stay whre it was, to care for the indigent, among other purposes.

Suspicions abounded anyhow: Hutchins would take the whole thing over, he didn't like doctors anyway, he was a dictator. Faculty members without tenure would be on their toes, the formidable A. J. (Ajax) Carlson, professor and chairman of physiology, was told by one of his colleagues supporting Hutchins. "You mean on their knees," he responded, meaning to the incumbent president.

The rumored merger, or "complete consolidation," as the *Chicago Times* reported in June of 1936, would be physical, in contrast to the mostly legal ties which made no day-to-day difference in students' lives. Up to half of them in any given year had no University of Chicago experience or loyalty anyhow.

By 1936 the university was ready to go it alone on the South Side. Rush submitted plans for a graduate program. But it was clear from these plans that Rush still wanted primarily to train practitioners. The university, on the other hand, wanted to advance medical science. This continued philosophical difference between the two institutions at least cooled university enthusiasm for a Rush graduate program.

In October of 1937, the university in effect gave Rush and Presbyterian five more years, at which point it would call a halt to its undergraduate involvement on the West Side. In June of 1938, what *The Chicago Herald-Examiner* called the "secession" question was discussed by both sides. Moving south ("Rush removal") was still a possibility. The advantages would be "closer association of scientific minds, elimination of overlapping departments and greater economy," according to Dr. Robert H. Herbst, retiring head of the Rush alumni association. Hutchins was "eager" for the move, some unidentified proponents said. Rush faculty and Presbyterian trustees were split on the question.

The faculty wanted to move. A faculty committee headed by Dr. Horace W. Armstrong reminded trustees that Presbyterian was "essentially a teaching hospital." Hutchins had already implied that the move to the South Side was the only solution, and the faculty committee understood that. Stay on the West Side, Armstrong said, and Rush had better look to Northwestern or the University of Illinois for a university affiliation.

Almost a year later, on June 1, 1939, 102 Rush faculty voted overwhelmingly to stay with the university, as opposed to shifting Rush affiliation to Northwestern for the sake of continued undergraduate teaching. They were split almost evenly in a subsequent mail ballot in the matter of "Rush removal" to the South Side. Eighty-five preferred to continue the connection by way of a West Side graduate program; 76 were willing to move south to keep the undergraduate program.

An alumnus who caught a reporter's ear cited familiar objections to moving: old-school ties and the complaint that on the South Side patient care was second to medical research. The university clinic patient, said the anonymous alumnus, was "just another experiment . . . a guinea pig." At "traditional schools like Rush," on the other hand, doctors were taught to feel "personal responsibility for their patients."

Reporting eight days later to the Presbyterian trustees, faculty spokesman Dr. George E. Shambaugh, Jr., argued for the graduate school solution. But Dr. Wilber Post, the Rush dean, argued for the move south. The proposed 300-bed South Side Presbyterian Hospital would cost only $3 million, he said, not the $4 million then projected, if the hospital would eliminate free beds and free outpatient service. This would make sense, he said, in view of coming national health and hospitalization insurance and expected loss of private donations. The Presbyterian endowment would subsidize research while patient care and clinical teaching paid for themselves, Post argued.

The Presbyterian trustees (more precisely, board of managers) were not convinced. The move south would cost too much and they were committed to the West Side. Three months later they voted to stay where they were and cooperate with the university in a graduate program.

In October of 1939, Hutchins, having been informed of their position, announced that the university would close Rush as an undergraduate school in 1942 and reopen it as a graduate school. Presbyterian board president John McKinlay announced at the same time that the hospital would stay where it was.

The Chicago Tribune reported the decision was made mostly because of expenses involved but also because of West Side clinical opportunities, which were considered more ample than those on the South Side.

At this point the university and Rush were still joined. But their union was headed for dissolution. In June of 1940, eight months after announcement of the decision to close the Rush undergraduate program, the divorce was also announced. Rush and the university would go their separate ways. Presbyterian Hospital (with Rush as a sort of alter ego) would affiliate with the University of Illinois.

This parting was friendly enough. The university returned everything it had acquired in the "final union" of 1924—even what had been added to the Rush endowment since then. Classes would be held for undergraduates during the coming year, after which no new students would be enrolled.

Hutchins said the problem had been the Rush faculty's insistence on continuing to do undergraduate teaching, followed by Presbyterian Hospital's refusal to come to the South Side. It had been agreed since 1916 that two undergraduate schools were out of the question and that Rush was to be a graduate school. Rush's decision to affiliate with the University of Illinois had finally ended the matter.

Some in the Rush camp, however, laid the problem at Hutchins' feet. He had wanted to close Rush down in any event, they claimed. He was not comfortable with privately practicing physicians as faculty members, referring to them as "quasi-faculty." He wanted everything on the South Side where he could control it.

Hutchins wore horns in the eyes of any number of people. But as Dwight Ingle observed in his sketch of Ajax Carlson, a critic of Hutchins, "In general, science flourished during his administration." So did Rush, up to a point.

Clinical Observations
1898–1946

THE GIANTS

When antimedicine evangelist John Alexander Dowie boldly invited Rush Medical College students to hear him lecture on "Drugs, Devils and Doctors" in the late 1890s, the students came in force, stank up the hall with a foul-smelling chemical and threw eggs at the man who had thrown down the gauntlet to them. It was not Rush's finest hour, though it did show school spirit of a sort.

Throwing eggs at Dowie was a bad idea. The students had better arguments against him in the persons of their teachers. There were giants in those days at Rush—Ludvig Hektoen, James B. Herrick, Frank Billings, Howard Taylor Ricketts, Arthur Bevan and Frederick Tice, to name a few. And there were giants yet to come—Bertram W. Sippy, Rollin Woodyatt, George and Gladys Dick and Dallas Phemister, all clinicians and researchers who strode the Rush, University of Chicago and Presbyterian and St. Luke's hospital corridors like colossi.

Hektoen, a pathologist, was Chicago's first medical scientist. A precise, charming man with a slight Norwegian accent, he was the first to say it mattered who gave blood to whom in the new field of blood transfusion and the first in Chicago, if not in the U.S., to make blood cultures from living patients. He helped produce measles in monkeys and discovered opsonin, a blood substance that helps leukocytes kill infection. He promoted autopsy as a research and teaching tool and performed the one in 1912 which James Herrick used as basis for his pioneering report on coronary thrombosis.

He and Herrick interned together at Cook County Hospital for 18 months beginning in April of 1888. Hektoen had been valedictorian of his class at the College of Physicians and Surgeons (later University of Illinois Medical School), Herrick of his at Rush. They had won their internships at County in competitive examinations, as was the rule in those days. Their friendship lasted 63 years, to Hektoen's death in 1951.

At County they had the good and bad experiences that went with working in that busy, beleaguered institution. Hektoen complained about rain leaking ''in torrents'' into the obstetrics ward, but he also worked under Senn and Fenger and finally chose pathology for his life work. In all, it was a heady experience.

He and Herrick left County after 18 months feeling they knew more than their peers who had interned elsewhere, more even than veterans—''old fogies''—who knew so little about bacteria, asepsis and the like. ''Bright young men of promise'' in their own eyes, Herrick wrote, in the eyes of others they may have been ''conceited upstarts.''

Hektoen joined Rush for a year as curator of its anatomy museum and lecturer in pathological anatomy and histology. In 1890 he became Chicago's first coroner's physician, lending credibility to that essentially political office. During the 1890s, he served also at his alma mater, the College of Physicians and Surgeons, and at Presbyterian, St. Luke's and County hospitals. In 10 years he published 30 papers. In the next 40 years, he published 270, winning for himself dozens of followers.

In 1902 he rejoined Rush and was, in addition, made head of the Memorial (later McCormick and yet later Hektoen) Institute for Infectious Diseases, and in 1904 became founding editor of *The Journal of Infectious Diseases*. In this capacity he became an expert, said Herrick, "at eliminating unnecessary words."

He held the Rush and McCormick Institute positions for more than 30 years. It almost was far less than that. Not long after he took them, he had an offer to teach at the University of Pennsylvania, at one of the nation's premier medical schools, but turned it down out of loyalty to Chicago.

The son of Norwegian Lutheran immigrants who became Wisconsin farmers, Hektoen had chosen medicine over theology. In his own life he combined intensity that sometimes flared into harshness with humility and a prankster's wit. "As a rule he was calm," Herrick wrote. But at least once he did not hold back and coauthored a book review that offended a Rush or university personage and almost cost him his job. The day and his job were saved when he apologized and showed that he hadn't written the offensive part.

Medical writer and Rush alumnus Dr. Morris Fishbein said Hektoen never showed pride except during a golf game when he sank a long putt. His pranksterism reportedly extended to the overnight feminization of a billboard bull across Harrison Street from County Hospital. Once he stationed an organ grinder on the sidewalk outside fellow pathologist Dr. E. R. LeCount's laboratory, where the man performed until paid to leave. To a prim colleague, he gave as a present a book dating from Elizabethan times using earthy Elizabethan language for body parts.

These were apparently part of his campaign against an over-hostile response to life's problems. Eventually, he learned to face life "with astonishing stoicism" and used his gift of humor to help others over hard spots. "But you don't itch!" he wrote Herrick in 1950, after Herrick had listed his many physical complaints in a note. The remark, like the man, was "laconic," noted Herrick the classicist—and yet "not only Spartan but Scandinavian" in its essence.

James Bryan Herrick was a suitable companion for Hektoen. He is known for two of the most famous achievements by the Rush-Presbyterian-University of Chicago staff in these years, the descriptions of coronary disease and of sickle-cell anemia—two otherwise unrelated pathologies.

He presented his sickle-cell discoveries in an article in November of 1910 in *The Archives of Internal Medicine,* where he described a patient of his and of Dr. Ernest Irons—a 20-year-old black man from Grenada, West Indies, who had been in the U.S. only three months. He had a chill, fever and headache and suffered from weakness and dizziness. His tongue was coated. He bore syphilis-like scars and had an enlarged heart with a "soft systolic murmur." The Wasserman test, for diagnosing syphilis, was negative. In the patient's blood, Herrick made "unusual findings."

Red corpuscles viewed under the microscope were of very irregular shape; many were thin, elongated, sickle-shaped and crescent-shaped. No parasites were found to account for any of this. The treatment was rest, good food and doses of syrup of iodide of iron. After four weeks the patient felt much better; some "sickling" remained, but it was not as noticeable. The ailment described here for the first time is what is now called sickle-cell anemia.

Others later identified the disease as inherited and chronic, chiefly among blacks. Pauling and others described the hemoglobin responsible for the condition. But Herrick's was the original description.

Herrick foreshadowed his second great discovery, a nuanced description of coronary artery thrombosis, in 1910 and 1911. But his 1912 article in *The Journal of the American Medical Association* is considered the first recognition of the disabling blockage of blood to the heart muscles known as myocardial infarction, or coronary thrombosis.

The coronary thrombosis had been described in the 1840s; most doctors thought it was inevitably fatal. But Herrick distinguished among occlusions (artery blockages) and thus arrived at a more hopeful outlook. Manifestations vary greatly, he said. He identified sufferers in whom the pain is great and symptoms recognizable, for whom the attack is usually fatal but not always and not immediately.

He warned against mistaking thrombosis for gall bladder disease, pancreatitis, hernia or other diseases and expressed his hope for development of a procedure of achieving adequate blood supply "through friendly neighboring vessels," which sounds a lot like bypass surgery. He showed that many victims can survive a heart attack and live useful lives if treated.

When Herrick read the 1912 paper before The Association of American Physicians, it "fell like a dud." But he "hammered away" at the topic in various forums for six years, until in 1918 he read another paper on the subject to the same group, and "the scales fell away from their eyes. . . . Physicians in America and later in Europe woke up and coronary thrombosis came into its own," he said. Herrick also, with Dr. Fred Smith, was the first to show a pattern of coronary blockage on an electrocardiograph machine.

After the 1912 article, he had to fight the term "heart specialist" for himself, because of its implication that he knew about nothing else. He knew about a lot else. Throughout his career, he dealt with all manner of medical problems. As an intern in 1888, he wrote about hemophilia, bladder rupture and tuberculosis. By 1954, when he died, he had written more than 160 articles on typhoid fever, leukemia, rheumatism, diabetes, pleurisy, gastric ulcer, gallstones, meningitis, malaria and many other subjects. Three articles he wrote for Sir William Osler's 1909 book, *Modern Medicine,* were about kidney disease.

As a clinician his experience was wide. He told an assistant how as a "heart specialist" he had that day discovered leukemia and several other ailments in four of six supposed heart patients. He was the first practitioner in Chicago to use the new diphtheria toxoid. Surgeons Senn, Murphy and Fenger relied on him, as later did Dean Lewis, Arthur Bevan and Vernon David. He was consultant of choice to the surgical giants of his day.

He possessed and cultivated what University of Chicago cardiologist Dr. Emmett Bay called "an absolute sense of touch," like the sense of pitch that a musician might have. "I would put a needle in there if I were you," he once said, pointing to the back of a patient whose problem had puzzled the Presbyterian Hospital staff for two weeks. They did as he directed and drew forth pus that hadn't shown on the X-ray.

He had an unusual ability to elicit a patient's history by questioning. Dr. Paul S. Rhoads, a Rush graduate and intern under Dr. George Dick at Presbyterian Hospital in the middle twenties, did an inadequate writeup of a patient for whom Herrick was called in to consult. Herrick sat down at bedside, questioned the patient and rewrote the history while Rhoads stood suffering in silence. Dick gave Rhoads a wink to show he knew what was happening. Herrick said not a word to the hapless intern, who learned this and other lessons well enough to be named distinguished Rush alumnus in 1979.

Herrick was a modest, almost shy man, careful about his appearance including the condition of his goatee. He and the husky, broad shouldered Dean Lewis were great friends. Lewis, for whom it was an especially proud moment when baseball star Ty Cobb consulted him about a sprained knee, took him to football games, where he explained things to the athletically untutored Herrick.

Among other giants was Dr. Frank Billings, whose focal infection theory remained a staple of medical practice for decades, though it was much abused and finally discarded. The theory was that chronic infection in one part of the body sometimes showed in other parts. Thus arthritis sometimes stemmed from infection in teeth or tonsils. Some practitioners carried the idea to extremes, needlessly removing teeth or tonsils. Billings also wrote extensively on arthritis and changes in the spinal cord during illness from pernicious anemia.

But he is known best as a fund raiser without equal—for Northwestern Medical School, The University of Chicago, Rush Medical College, Presbyterian Hospital, the McCormick Institute, Provident Hospital and probably a dozen other causes. In his philanthropic efforts he did not hesitate to call on relatives who walked in the first ranks of Chicago entrepreneurs. One of them, his uncle, Albert Merritt Billings, headed People's Gas Light and Coke Company for many years. The University of Chicago hospital was named after him.

Born on a Wisconsin farm in 1854, Frank Billings attended Chicago Medical College and interned at County Hospital. He returned to teach at his alma mater, left for European studies, returned to teach again at Chicago Medical College (now Northwestern University Medical School), and in 1898 joined Rush, where he became dean of the faculty. Shrewd and able to "pull wires," he had a "genius for leadership" which enabled him, in Herrick's phrase, to plan and "push plans through."

He organized doctors to form a professional office complex on the 14th floor of the People's Gas Building on Michigan Avenue. Many Presbyterian and St. Luke's Hospital staff members, years before the merger of these two institutions, officed there. The 14th floor became the place to go for treatment by the city's medical elite.

A genial, sympathetic man who "radiated the impression of power," Billings had an infectious sense of humor. Herrick called him "a rare personality" who "attracted people by his big frame, his strong face, and his evident sincerity of purpose." He was "forceful, often aggressive, intensely human, with strong likes and dislikes, even inconsistencies" but "did not cringe or fawn before wealth, title or social position, nor did he shrink from poverty or ignorance." Among his trainees he counted some of the city's leading medical and surgical lights, including Doctors Ernest Irons, Joseph Miller, Joseph Capps and Wilber Post.

He died in 1932, widely mourned. His colleagues Herrick, Post and Vernon David praised the "moral factor" that dominated his activities, drew others to him, inspired them to do their best and "created high morale in the institutions where he worked."

Another notable performer was Dr. Frederick Tice, a Rush alumnus who for years was Chicago's leading authority on tuberculosis. He was medical superintendent at County Hospital, taught at the College of Physicians and Surgeons and at

Rush and opened one of the city's first tuberculosis clinics. Later he became president of the Municipal Tuberculosis Sanitarium.

Tice was also notable for the 10-volume, loose-leaf encyclopedia of medical practice which he started in 1915. Its special value lay in the way it could be regularly brought up to date by publication of new loose-leaf pages.

Dr. Arthur Dean Bevan, Rush teacher and Presbyterian staff member, was a major figure especially because of his work on the 1910 study of U.S. medical education known as the Flexner Report. As a surgeon, Bevan pioneered the use of ethylene-oxygen as an anesthetic, an area in which he and his friend Arno Luckhardt did research.

Bevan's connection with the Flexner Report in essence began in 1905, when the American Medical Association's Council on Medical Education, which Bevan chaired, singled out five states ("especially rotten spots") responsible for "most of the [country's] bad medical instruction." One of them was Illinois; of its 54 medical schools, at most six were "acceptable" to the council.

This almost blanket condemnation led eventually to funding by the Carnegie Foundation in 1909 of the study by Abraham Flexner, an educator chosen partly because he lacked medical background and thus presumably would bring a fresh approach to the problem. Flexner's report, published the following year, echoed the comments by the AMA committee that Bevan had headed, harshly criticizing medical education in the U.S. and Canada.

This is not surprising, since Flexner was acting as unannounced surrogate for the AMA, which wanted to attack without being attacked. In Illinois only three institutions—Rush, Northwestern and the College of Physicians and Surgeons (later University of Illinois)—made the cut. Rush made it because of its recently raised admission standards and its facilities and scientific work, which Flexner rated tops in the state.

Flexner had toured 155 schools, including 34 in six states during a one-month "meteoric dash" in April of 1909. He decided only 35 of the 155 were needed. Bevan downgraded the report before a Chicago audience but later endorsed it. He didn't admit AMA involvement in the study until 1928.

Apart from his kind words for Rush's standards and laboratories, Flexner was hard on the place, calling it "a divided school" whose two branches, one on the West Side, one on the South, did not form "an organic whole." Presbyterian Hospital he said was "not by any means a genuine teaching hospital," which may or may not have reflected Bevan's thoughts about his own institutions.

At those institutions Bevan was a hard taskmaster, training many surgeons, including Dallas Phemister, who later was head of surgery at Billings Hospital and himself trained a number of outstanding surgeons. Bevan "gave every man of promise a square deal and the opportunity to make good," in Herrick's words.

Even in his 70s, Bevan remained a master surgeon, operating with almost no bleeding. He worked fast and well and was a "gentle, superb and technical operator," according to Dr. R. Kennedy Gilchrist, who was an intern at the time.

Dr. Bertram W. Sippy gained fame through his treatment of peptic ulcers, as by use of "Sippy powder," and by his quantitative analysis of a patient's gastric content. One of his great achievements was to teach patients how to measure and control their own acidity. Patients would remain hospitalized for up to six weeks, regularly extracting material from within themselves for testing.

Sippy would discuss a patient's condition with patient and numerous staff present for as long as 45 minutes, so absorbed was he in his subject. He was well liked anyhow, in spite of his "garrulity, needless repetition of medical truisms and lack of promptness," said Herrick.

THE INSTITUTIONS

Dr. Francis Straus recalls having his adenoids removed at Presbyterian Hospital in 1901 when he was six years old. Arriving by train from his suburban home, he was taken to a second-floor corner room in the Jones Building where coals burned in an open fireplace. From there he was taken to the operating room, where he inhaled ethyl bromide as an anesthetic. It was considered potentially fatal at the time, he learned years later. The operation finished, he was taken the same day in a hansom cab to catch the Burlington Railroad train back home.

Seven years later, Straus, who later taught at Rush and was on the Presbyterian staff, might have been put up in the new Private Pavilion adjoining Jones, built in 1908 mainly for use by private patients. This pavilion was built only after the hospital's medical board practically guaranteed its economic viability to the board of managers, promising that as an investment its $300,000 cost would outperform bonds and mortgages. Thus paying patients would subsidize charity patients.

Four years later, Presbyterian built the Jane Murdock Memorial Building for women and children, which partly replaced the original Ross and Hamill wings. Its $175,000 cost had been willed for the purpose by the late Thomas Murdock. The Jones Memorial was later remodeled and expanded, so that by 1922 the hospital had room for 435 patients.

The Memorial Institute for Infectious Diseases was founded in 1902 in memory of John Rockefeller McCormick, the son of Harold F. and Edith Rockefeller McCormick, who donated the money for it at the urging of Frank Billings after their son died of scarlet fever. In 1918 it was renamed the John McCormick Institute for Infectious Diseases and in 1943 renamed again the Hektoen Institute for Medical Research. It was at first quartered in the Rush laboratory building at 1743 West Harrison Street.

Operated under direction of the institute was the 40-bed Anna W. Durand Hospital, where sufferers from diphtheria, scarlet fever, measles and other infectious diseases were cared for without charge. Durand opened in 1913 in its own building at Wood and Flournoy streets under Dr. George H. Weaver as director. A connecting institute laboratory opened in 1914 just north of it on Wood Street. Each building was four stories. The hospital also had a sun room and roof garden.

Bedside instruction was given to groups of three to five Rush students in the Durand wards. Students wore caps and gowns to protect against infection. Each carefully washed his or her hands after touching anything in the patient's vicinity. The precautions were successful; no students were known to become infected.

Rush faculty and students were closely associated with both institute and hospital. Rush provided many young men and women willing to work at both places, which in turn provided clinical material and helped Rush maintain its atmosphere of research.

An example of the research was a description by Dr. Stanton A. Friedberg, Sr., in 1916 in *The Journal of the American Medical Association* of removal of tonsils as neutralizer of the diphtheria carrier. The carrier would infect others though not infected with diphtheria. Dr. Friedberg's son, Stanton A., Jr., also a distinguished otolaryngologist at Presbyterian and Presbyterian–St. Luke's hospitals, was medical staff president from 1964 to 1966.

As director of the institute, Hektoen supervised and contributed substantially to the studies of scarlet fever by Dr. George Dick and his wife, Gladys Henry Dick, who together found its cause and devised a test for susceptibility to it and an antitoxin for treatment of it.

Contemporary with McCormick-Durand was the Otho S. A. Sprague Memorial Institute founded in 1911 by Rush trustee Albert A. Sprague with funds from the estate of his late brother Otho S. A. Sprague. The Spragues were in the wholesale food business, under the company name of Sprague-Warner. They had already contributed to the Presbyterian Hospital nursing school building.

The Sprague Institute built no buildings but supported research at The University of Chicago and at Rush, Presbyterian, Children's Memorial, St. Luke's and Cook County hospitals, with emphasis on discovering chemical solutions to medical problems. University of Chicago pathologist Dr. H. Gideon Wells was its first director. Like McCormick-Durand it became part of the 1916 plan for the university's medical school.

By the early twenties, half of the 20-member Sprague professional staff worked full time for the institute. James Herrick headed its advisory council, which included pathologists Hektoen and E. R. LeCount and internist Billings, who also headed its trustees. Among these were Albert A. Sprague II and Martin Ryerson, president of The University of Chicago board of trustees.

Sprague Institute work included search for a safe antituberculosis drug and work on rheumatism and diabetes. Billings headed the rheumatism work in specially designated Presbyterian Hospital wards. Dr. Rollin Woodyatt led the diabetes research.

Sprague-sponsored work also took place at Children's Memorial Hospital, which was affiliated with Rush from 1910 to 1919. Rush faculty not only supervised the teaching at Children's but staffed and ran the place, which had room for about 30 patients and a small outpatient department. Various additions expanded capacity to 150 patients by the early twenties, including contagious ones. In 1919 Children's transferred its affiliation to The University of Chicago in anticipation of the coming South Side medical school.

In spite of Rush's research orientation, the college was accused in 1917 of shirking its academic responsibilities and turning out mere practitioners. Rush graduates knew no more about current medical experimentation than would a ''clubwoman in three weeks reading for a 'paper,' '' editorialized *The University of Chicago Magazine.*

H. Gideon Wells, director of the Sprague Institute, could not let this pass. ''Nothing could be farther from the truth,'' he responded. The emphasis at Rush was on investigation in a graduate school atmosphere, he said. Rush students, moreover, regularly published in various journals, including *The Journal of the American Medical Association.* Actually, Wells wrote, the usual complaint was the opposite, that Rush made its students investigators, not physicians. Wells said he found ''balm'' in the magazine's allegation. ''Perhaps we are doing something to make doctors after all,'' he said.

The Rush program for making doctors included ''ward courses'' for small groups of seniors three hours a day for one quarter at Presbyterian. Some students took "extramural" courses, not supervised by Rush faculty, at the West Side Hebrew Dispensary and at Alexian Brothers, St. Anthony's and St. Luke's hospitals.

In general the many options for clinical work at Rush gave it major appeal and helped to draw medical students to The University of Chicago. The pathologist LeCount, for instance, was doing thousands of autopsies and was a first-rate pedagog besides. He would ask a student to look at a piece of tissue, and then cover it with his hands and ask the student what he saw. If the student began to describe what was covered, as most did, he was in trouble. What LeCount wanted to hear was what the student saw (the hand), not what was covered. It was a test of hearing what was asked and no more and answering that alone.

Presbyterian Hospital itself was controlled in medical matters by the Rush faculty, who staffed it. The superintendent of Presbyterian in the early part of the century, Dr. Henry B. Stehman, retired in 1906. Many of his duties fell to a former clerk who had developed a talent for innovation in what was then a new field. This was Asa Bacon, a protégé of the first president of the hospital's board of managers, Dr. D. K. Pearsons.

Bacon is credited with creating the concept of training courses for hospital administrators and running the first one in 1907. In the same year, he founded and became first president of the Chicago Cook County Hospital Association. Plans for hospital construction that he developed in 1916, considered revolutionary at the time, later became common practice.

Stehman's successor as president of Presbyterian was Albert M. Day, a retired businessman who knew little about hospitals but did well as a fund raiser.

The Presbyterian Hospital School of Nursing was established in 1903. Its nurse training had been done by the Illinois Training School for Nurses. The first director, M. Helena McMillan, was one of only four in its 53 years. She served to 1938. Persuaded by her father not to pursue a doctor's career, she acquired a bachelor of arts degree from McGill University (far above nursing standards of the day) and studied at the Illinois Training School.

A generous, determined woman with a sense of humor, Miss McMillan pretty much created the Presbyterian school, which was one of the first to put its students on an eight-hour day and one of the first to charge tuition. Its course of three and a half years was longer than most schools, and it was affiliated with a medical school, Rush, whose clinics provided good learning experience. Unlike many schools, its classes were held in the daytime and nurses lived close by.

The first nurses' residence was a former girls' club at 277 South Ashland Avenue, at Congress Street. After 1912 nurses lived at the Sprague Home, at 1750 West Congress Street, across from the hospital.

Incoming Presbyterian students were told to bring four gingham or calico dresses and "noiseless shoes." Students wore a pin with "PHSN" engraved on it, not a cross, as most nursing students wore. The cap, which sat on the back of the head, was simple, without folds and tucks, and kept the nurse's hair out of the way.

Early lecturers in the nursing school included Billings, Herrick, Bevan, and LeCount. In 1907 obstetrics training was moved to the Lying-In Hospital, and pediatrics to the Jackson Park Baby Sanitarium. There was also pediatrics at Presbyterian, headed in the twenties by Dr. Clifford Grulee.

Other clinical learning opportunities were offered by the Home for Destitute Crippled Children, at Washington Boulevard and Paulina Street on the West Side. Rush conducted teaching clinics in orthopedic surgery and other subjects at the Home, which was a short walk away.

Presbyterian Hospital received Chicago's first electrocardiograph in 1913, 10 years after it was developed as a practical device for recording heart activity. It was the gift (through Dr. James Herrick, who used it to track coronary thrombosis) of Nettie McCormick, widow of Cyrus.

In 1921 Rush opened a five-room children's clinic at the Central Free Dispensary, with kindergarten-style tables and chairs in its waiting area. This was the first section of the dispensary set aside for children, though 500 children a month were seen there. That number was sure to rise, dispensary superintendent Gertrude Howe Britton told a reporter.

Medicine in general in the early twenties had its own flavor and ambience. Its appeal to ambitious young men was limited, for one thing, as a Yale graduate of the time recalled in 1977. He is Dr. Samuel G. Taylor III, an oncologist who was director of the Illinois Cancer Council and helped start the Rush Cancer Center.

Most of Taylor's class at Yale went on to Wall Street to make money. Medical schools did not require top grades. Once in the trenches, as it were, as when Taylor interned at County Hospital, one found the chief killer was pneumonia, which had an 80 percent mortality rate. Syphilis was common and treatable only in the early stages. Scarlet fever and erysipelas cases crowded the contagious wards. Cerebral damage from whooping cough and measles encephalitis were also common.

A few miles to the east, at St. Luke's Hospital, Doctors Casey Wood and Frank Allport opened an eye, ear, nose and throat clinic about 1910. An outpatient division was opened in 1917.

In the twenties, half the St. Luke's staff had teaching appointments at Northwestern Medical School, the rest at the University of Illinois. Many St. Luke's doctors also served at Northwestern-affiliated Passavant Hospital.

St. Luke's had 400 beds in 1923 and was caring for more than 9,800 patients a year. Costs of non-paying patients were covered by users of the George Smith Memorial Building. St. Luke's, though founded by members of the Episcopal Church, was "in no sense a sectarian institution" and practiced "no discrimination as to race or creed," according to a fund raising brochure. The fund raising was successful. The Indiana Avenue building went up, and by 1930 St. Luke's had reached a capacity of 697 beds.

The twenties were distinguished by yet another, more auspicious St. Luke's Hospital event with the advent in 1927 of the annual Woman's Board fashion show, which by the mid-fifties was raising more than $50,000 a year and by the mid-eighties was raising many times that amount.

DOCTORS, NURSES, PATIENTS

In the early thirties, there were 25 applicants for each internship at Presbyterian Hospital. The heavy patient load was the main attraction, since other aspects of the assignment were anything but engaging. The intern was given room and board and had his laundry done for him but was paid nothing. He even bought his own uniform. Now and then he could pick up a few dollars for a pint of his blood. Otherwise, he was on his own.

One of the "services" in which he might work for three months or so at a time was with Dr. George Dick of scarlet fever fame, who was to leave for Billings Hospital on the South Side in July of 1932. Dick and his wife, Gladys, had isolated the scarlet fever organism and produced an immunizing serum. He was a big quiet fellow, well over six feet tall and bald, with expressive eyes and a sense of humor.

He was a very good teacher, "one of the few who really made one think," according to R. K. Gilchrist, one of his interns. If an intern asked him something he could have learned from a textbook, Dick wouldn't answer him. But if Dick realized the intern had looked it up first and still had a question, he would give the young man or woman 15 minutes of his time while standing in a stairwell or wherever else the question was asked.

A pathologist, he taught students to "think disease," a skill more important in the days before laboratory tests played their all-important role. That is, students were to take a patient's history, examine, take blood counts and blood pressure and do urine analyses staying ever alert to identifying the problem.

Another "service" was under the distinguished Dr. Kellogg Speed, former University of Chicago football star, English scholar and war hero. When Speed gave his course on fractures at County Hospital, guards had to be posted to make sure Rush students got their half of the amphitheatre seats, such was Speed's popularity.

Another service was with Dr. Rollin T. Woodyatt, the world famous diabetes specialist. Woodyatt was the first to use insulin in Chicago and in the thirties at Presbyterian was teaching children as young as five years old how to give themselves insulin. He and a biochemist, Dr. E. J. Witzemann, produced insulin at Rush. Woodyatt was a nephew of the famed city planner Daniel Burnham.

Dr. Herman Kretschmer, later president of the AMA, had another service. Kretschmer was a shrewd diagnostician who gave two or three blood transfusions a day of whole, uncitrated resident blood which worked wonders, passing on antibodies and the like where they could do the most good.

Among nurses at Presbyterian were endowed nurses, specialists who cared for the indigent. These were widely used during these years, beginning with the first such endowment in 1917. Endowed nurses were known by the name of the person in whose honor the endowment was given. Thus there were Helen North Nurses, Gladys Foster Nurses, Ernest A. Hamill Nurses, etc.

The floors at Presbyterian were designated by letters—A floor, B floor, etc. The head nurse on D floor and trainer of many nurses, a woman named Dessie Greek, had served during the Great War with the 13th Army Base Hospital, staffed by the Presbyterian-Rush contingent, and had not forgotten what she learned of military discipline.

She kept her floor sparkling clean and enforced regulations to the letter unless a patient belonged to the American Legion, in which case special attention would be paid. She also was not above (or below) ordering up scrambled eggs from the diet kitchen for a surgeon and his resident whom she met in the midst of their rounds.

Nurses and doctors then as now often married each other. Nurses were forbidden to marry while in training, however, whether doctors or anyone else, though some did and kept it secret. Many married once the course was complete.

Durand Hospital was the scene of sometimes heroic efforts to save children choking to death from laryngeal diphtheria. They would be brought in at all hours, their chests heaving, gasping for air that could not make it past the diphtheric membrane formed in the windpipe. A big fire gong would go off at the foot of a resident's bed on the fifth (top) floor. He would jump up, put on pants and slippers and hit the floor running.

A nurse would meet him at the top of the stairs with a gown, cap and mask which he donned in seconds. He was with the patient almost immediately, slipping a rubber tube into the trachea, if necessary through a metal one inserted first. Nurses would slip in a mouth gag to keep the child from biting the doctor as the two engaged in their life-and-death struggle. Then the blocking membrane would be sucked out. R. K. Gilchrist, whose recollections these are, did 20 such "intubations" in his first three weeks at Durand, where he spent three months. After that he lost track.

Diagnoses in those days were made without expensive testing and relied heavily on the doctor's experience. When a needle inserted into the chest of a moderately sick patient drew out "brick red fluid," for instance, the examining physician might spot the problem immediately as an amoebic abscess of the liver that had broken through the diaphragm.

Presbyterian Hospital, being on Chicago's West Side, had its dealings with the crime syndicate. Al Capone's successor as syndicate chief, Frank Nitti, known as "The Enforcer," a little dark-haired man, was a patient. So was another syndicate member whom Dr. Ernest Irons treated, without knowing the man's provenance. In gratitude, the man threw a party for Irons and gave him a watch, which later checked out as worth a paltry $15.

Dr. Vernon David operated on the syndicate's slot-machine chief, Eddie Vogel, under an alias—Vogel's, not David's. Later a syndicate lawyer sent a scrubwoman to be treated for skin cancer and, in Robin Hood style, paid her bill. Gilchrist later, knowing nothing about the man's clients, begged $200 from him to fund a research project.

Others gave and raised money from a different background —the women's auxiliaries or boards of Presbyterian and St. Luke's hospitals. The president of the St. Luke's Woman's Board from 1926 to 1944, Mrs. John W. Gary, presided at meetings in no-nonsense fashion. She and the other older members sat at a long table, she at one end and Mrs. Walter

B. Wolf, who later succeeded her, at the other. The younger women sat along the wall.

It was at the start of Mrs. Gary's incumbency that two Woman's Board members, Mrs. Hathaway Watson and Mrs. Frank Hibbard, suggested an annual fund raising fashion show. The two had seen charity fashion shows in France, one in Deauville and the other in Cannes. Together they decided that what was good for Deauville and Cannes was good for Chicago. The elegant, popular event became an institution.

The first show was held at the Stevens (later Hilton) Hotel on October 27, 1927. Afternoon and dinner shows were held with a tea in between. After some years at the Stevens, shows were held at Orchestra Hall and, since 1945, the Medinah Temple.

Mrs. Clyde E. Shorey was president of the Presbyterian Hospital Woman's Board in the mid-thirties (1936–1938) and early forties (1941–1945) and dedicated herself unstintingly to its success over several ensuing decades. She died in 1984 in her 90s.

Those who served the St. Luke's Woman's Board in the forties and fifties included Mrs. Gordon Lang, Mrs. Eric Oldberg, Mrs. Robert McCormick Adams, Mrs. Charles H. Morse, Jr., and Mrs. Fentress Ott. Working with the board in its various ventures were Leo Lyons, director of St. Luke's Hospital from 1942 to 1956, and Cornelia Conger, its decorator, who bought all the hospital's china and decorated its rooms, leaning often on Woman's Board members for guidance.

At the two hospitals during these years, including the early forties, several health care milestones were passed. During 1932, for instance, the Presbyterian-Rush staff-faculty performed 75 cornea transplants. During the same year, only a few were done elsewhere in the U.S.

Dr. Eric Oldberg's successful performance of brain surgery in 1933 was among the first done in that field. St. Luke's opened Chicago's first audiology service in 1937. Presbyterian offered such a service in the early fifties. Also in the thirties, the new psychiatric unit at St. Luke's was another first for a private hospital in the U.S.

THE TWO WARS

The two world wars involved staffs of both hospitals. The first Presbyterian staff person to enter service in the first war was the nurse in charge of outpatient service, Alma Foerster, who enlisted in the fall of 1914 with the American Red Cross for service in Russia. She later served in Rumania and was decorated by both these countries and by the Red Cross.

One who left shortly after her was Serbian-born Dr. John M. Kara, who died of typhus fever while on duty with the Serbian army medical corps. The epidemic in which he died was finally brought under control with delousing methods based on the findings of another Rush teacher, the medical martyr Dr. Howard Taylor Ricketts.

Ricketts had died five years earlier in Mexico working on a cure for typhus, which he discovered was transmitted by lice. Hence the delousing, which in Serbia and elsewhere saved thousands of lives. Ricketts had already done extensive work on Rocky Mountain or tick fever in Idaho and on blastomycotic (fungus) infection of the skin.

Foerster and Kara were the first of dozens of Rush and Presbyterian personnel who went to war, almost all in medical service. The 13th U.S. Army Base Hospital was organized at Presbyterian in the fall of 1916. Dr. Frank Billings, dean of the Rush faculty, was its commanding officer. But Billings caught a near fatal pneumonia and was replaced by Dr. Arthur Bevan.

Others on the staff of the 13th were Dr. Dean D. Lewis, of the department of surgery; Dr. Basil C. H. Harvey, professor of anatomy and later dean of students on the South Side medical campus; and Dr. Ralph C. Brown, of the department of medicine. The unit entered service in January of 1918 at Camp Jackson, Mississippi, and left for Europe in April. It served to the war's end in November.

In the summer of 1917, Billings headed an American Red Cross mission to Russia to survey conditions there. Dr. Wilber Post joined him on this mission, which lasted two months. Just after the war, Dr. H. Gideon Wells headed a similar relief mission for the U.S. Army to Rumania. Post was also part of a four-month relief mission to Persia in 1918 headed by University of Chicago President Harry P. Judson.

Dozens of Rush faculty helped at ROTC camps. Fifteen Rush graduates took Navy medical commissions. Seventy of the Rush junior class signed as nonmedical personnel in the 13th, and over 60 sophomores joined an ambulance corps organized by Captain Elbert Clark, of the department of anatomy. Most of these dropout volunteers later withdrew to stay in medical school, heeding an urgent government plea to do so.

The Medical Enlisted Reserve Corps., composed of medical students who belonged to the Army, was formed in August of 1917. The entire Rush-University of Chicago Medical School student body began studying on both campuses under military command, living in barracks opposite Hull Laboratories on the South Side and in the West Side YMCA on Monroe Street on the West Side.

They wore uniforms for the few months that remained of the war and drilled three times a week on the former Chicago Cubs baseball field two blocks south of Rush.

In all, 100 or so of the Rush-University of Chicago faculty served in the Medical Corps, many overseas in the hospital at Limoges, France. Seventy-five others served in other ways. Both South and West Side campuses remained open at full capacity.

The St. Luke's staff formed the 14th Field Hospital together with the staff of Michael Reese Hospital. Dr. L. L. McArthur and nurse Ellen Stewart organized it, but neither could accompany it overseas. Instead, Dr. Samuel Plummer, a St. Luke's surgeon, and Mrs. Lynnette L. Vandervort, a nurse who later won a Distinguished Service Medal, headed the unit when it went to France. Fifty of the unit's nurses were from St. Luke's, 50 from Reese. Activated in the fall of 1917, it went first to camps in this country, where pneumonia and contagious diseases had to be fought in barracks conditions and without the help of sulfa and penicillin.

The unit later paraded in New York City before sailing in

July of 1918 for Liverpool, which it reached on August 11. Some of its members served in Paris, others on the English coast in an early Elizabethan house from which they could see France on a clear day. The old house was loaned by its owner, Sir Arthur Markham, who also donated an X-ray and ambulance. Lady Markham, his wife, did most of the cooking for staff and patients. The house-hospital had beds for 50 and an operating room. More primitive conditions prevailed in Belgium, where some of the war wounded had to undergo amputations without anesthetic, according to one account.

In World War II, Presbyterian and St. Luke's doctors and nurses served again in the 13th and 14th Army hospital units, though not all. The Presbyterian unit began recruiting in 1942, thanks largely to Dr. L. C. Gatewood, a veteran of the Presbyterian unit in the first war, who had remained in contact with the War Department.

The 13th's doctors and nurses were recruited with ease almost entirely from Presbyterian. The unit offered the doctor a way out of being drafted, which was universally considered a bad way to enter the Army even by those who were willing to go. The Army would use doctors as it wished in any event, removing them from this unit as they were needed elsewhere —to head other units, for instance. This World War II unit was a general hospital, not a base hospital, as was the one in World War I.

Recruiting for enlisted men was harder, but the quota was filled by October of 1942. Once formed, the unit met several nights a week on the South and West sides for drilling and lectures. In December the first cadre was inducted and sent to Camp Grant near Rockford, Illinois. From there they were off to Camp Robinson, near Little Rock. In all, the unit numbered 20 or so doctors, almost 100 nurses and 350 enlisted men —plumbers, barbers, carpenters and the like. Among the doctors were Edwin Miller, the unit's chief of surgery, Evan Barton, R. K. Gilchrist, Holmes Nicoll, Francis Straus and George Stuppy.

Many Presbyterian nursing students joined the U.S. Cadet Nurse Corps during these years. The cadet program, 1943 to

1948, marked the first underwriting by the federal government of nursing education. It was also the first time nursing classes were offered at Presbyterian on a racially and religiously non-discriminatory basis.

The 13th hospital left Little Rock in May for the Desert Training Center at Spadra, California, a camp in the desert near Los Angeles, where they pitched tents and dug in to care for those injured in nearby desert maneuvers. Wooden barracks, hot water and other amenities eventually replaced the tents.

In September they went to Utah, and in January of 1944 they left on a converted Dutch liner for New Zealand, Australia and finally New Guinea. In New Guinea, they set up a general hospital 60 miles behind the lines to receive casualties from station hospitals. In the early weeks in this jungle location, dysentery and skin diseases, such as jungle rot, were a regular concern.

In May of 1945, Evan Barton, who had headed the unit's laboratory service, was made commanding officer. In June the unit was off to the Philippines, in October to Japan. By December of 1946, when the unit was officially deactivated, most had gone home.

Not all Rush-Presbyterian doctors went with the 13th. A group was taken from it while in Australia and sent to form the second and 25th portable surgical hospitals. This was eventually commanded by Dr. Frederic de Peyster (later Major), a 1940 Rush graduate. As part of the 32nd Infantry, the 25th saw action on a series of Pacific islands, including Okinawa, Ie Shima (where correspondent Ernie Pyle was killed by a sniper's bullet), and the Philippines. On September 6, 1945, after the Japanese surrender, the 32nd entered southern Japan, where de Peyster's portable hospital group set up the first American hospital. Every doctor but one in the 25th was a Rush graduate.

Presbyterian's doctors for the most part stayed together during the war, but St. Luke's did not. Some served in North Africa and Italy with the 14th General Hospital, setting up hospitals in Naples and then in France. In the one in France, there was one nurse to every 100 patients and the staff performed 60 to 90 operations a day.

Others, 35 of them, joined the Army Air Corps after the Army and Navy told Dr. Foster McMillan they weren't needed. McMillan finally went to Washington, where he found the Air Corps needed them very much. St. Luke's had two Air Corps units, one headed by McMillan and Dr. John Brewer, the other by Dr. Marvin Flannery. The first went to Denver, to set up Buckley Hospital, near Buckley Field.

The other went to Amarillo, Texas, though later Brewer went to Amarillo too, to head the hospital there. Doctors Ormand Julian and Earl Merz (later head of ophthalmology at Northwestern) were in the Amarillo group. In general the St. Luke's men were split off from the original St. Luke's group as the Air Corps found other posts for them.

Back on the home front at Presbyterian, nonprofessional volunteers were trained to help the short-handed staff, including a contingent of male Wilson & Company employees in 1944. Women volunteers came from the Red Cross and from the ranks of the Woman's Board. Mrs. Clyde Shorey headed the latter group. It was the first time direct service for patients —taking temperatures, for instance—was performed by volunteers. A bright spot in the middle of the war was the bequest to the hospital of $450,000 from the estate of the widow of Dr. Arthur Bevan.

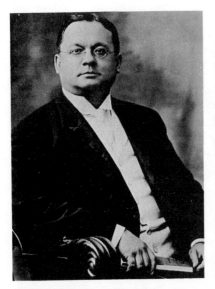

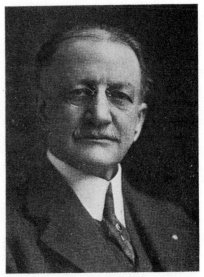

William Rainey Harper,
1856–1906, founder of
The University of Chicago.
(Photo courtesy University of Chicago)

E. Fletcher Ingals, M.D.,
1848–1918.

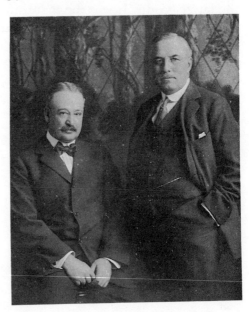

Frank Billings, M.D.,
1854–1932, and Arthur
Dean Bevan, M.D.,
1861–1943.

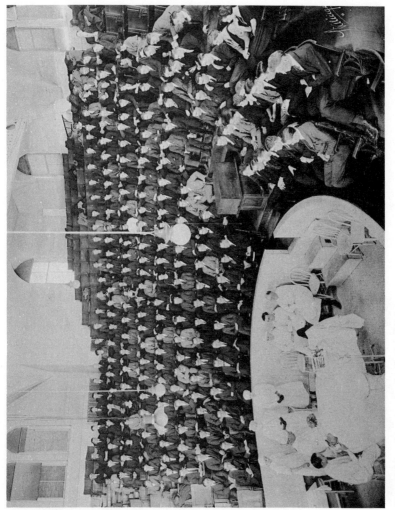

Dr. Bevan's surgical clinic, 1925.

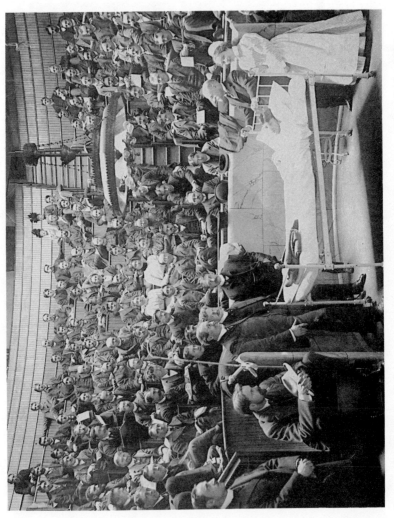

James B. Herrick, M.D., conducted clinics at Cook County Hospital, 1900.

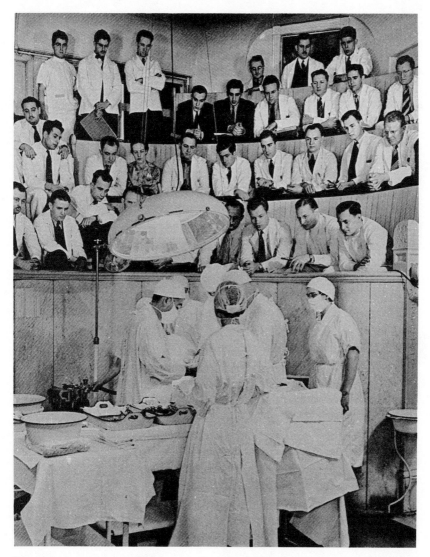

Teaching surgery, 1938.

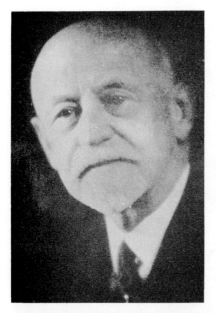

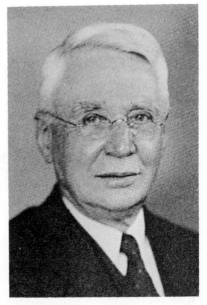

James B. Herrick, M.D.
1861–1954.

Ludvig Hektoen, M.D.
1863–1951.

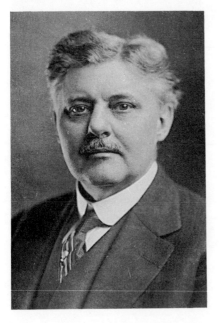

Bertram W. Sippy, M.D.
1866–1924.

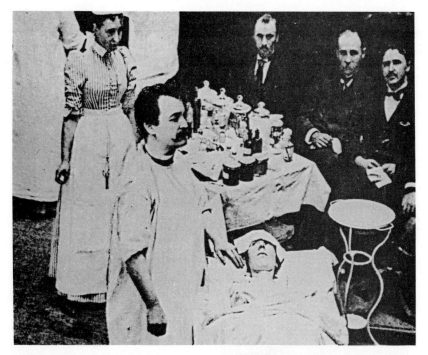

Nicholas Senn, M.D., conducts surgery clinic in amphitheatre of
Rush Medical College.

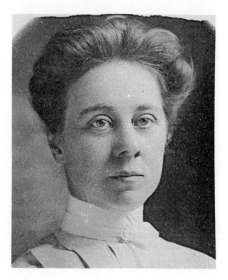

M. Helena McMillan, R.N.
1868–1970, founder of
Presbyterian Hospital School
of Nursing in 1903.

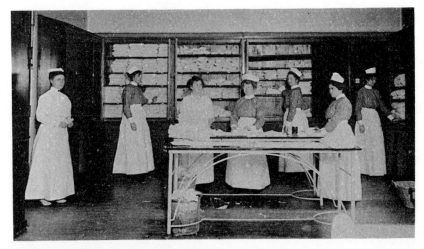

Surgical supplies room, Presbyterian Hospital, 1910.

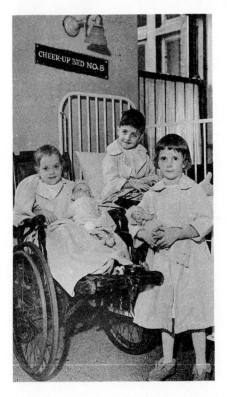

Children's Ward,
Presbyterian Hospital,
1937.

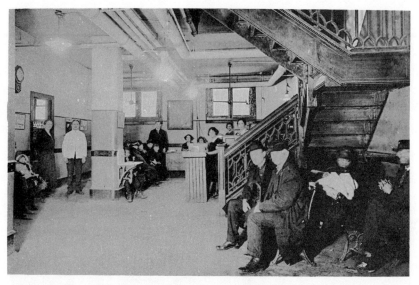

Central Free Dispensary waiting room, 1923.

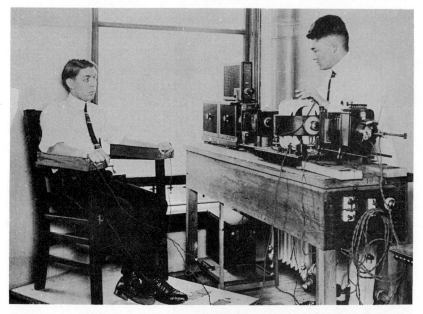

First electrocardiogram at Rush Medical College/Presbyterian Hospital, 1913.

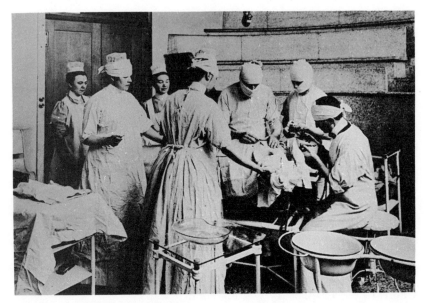

St. Luke's Hospital operating room, 1913.

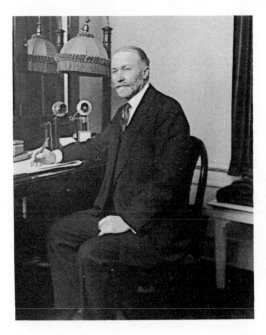

John Benjamin Murphy,
M.D., 1857–1916.
(Courtesy Mercy Hospital of Chicago)

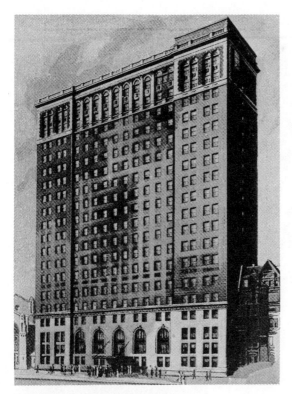

St. Luke's Hospital, 1925.

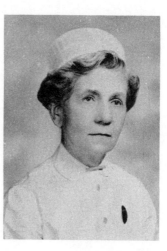

Madeleine McConnell, R.N.,
1888–1983.

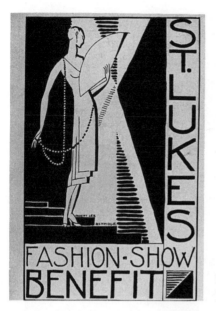

Poster for Woman's Board
Fashion Show in 1927.

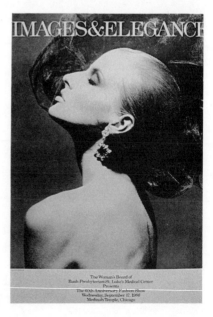

Fashion Show Poster, 1986.

Postwar Revival
1946–1955

At Presbyterian Hospital in 1946, the mood was shaped by two major events of the past five years, the war just ended and the split with The University of Chicago. The war had been disruptive, of course. Doctors and nurses left. Supplies and services were short. The hospital functioned short-handed. Life went on but with a sometimes grim expectancy. At the same time, there was a huge, unprecedented governmental involvement in medical matters which was to make a great difference to Presbyterian.

The split with the university was disrupting, as was the simultaneous mothballing of Rush Medical College. For the first time in its almost 60 years, the hospital had gone it alone without Rush. The Presbyterian staff was adjusting to its new identity.

The hospital affiliated with The University of Illinois in 1941, the year the Chicago Medical Center District was created by the state legislature and given power to buy and clear slum land. Presbyterian and The University of Illinois were in the district. So were Cook County Hospital and its

121

affiliates, the Loyola University and Chicago Medical schools and some state laboratories. Presbyterian might have felt orphaned, but its West Side location was receiving a powerful boost from government.

The Presbyterian-University of Illinois agreement preserved the independence of each. The hospital pledged cooperation with the university, which was to have access to the hospital's facilities. Neither institution assumed budgetary obligations for the other.

Hospital appointments were to be made by hospital trustees after a process of nomination and approval by the university. This nomination process has been commonly thought to have given the university veto power, never exercised, over hospital appointments, but it didn't quite say that.

Furthermore, the university was to appoint the hospital staff to its own clinical staff (would "blanket" them in, as one veteran put it) and was free to nominate "a limited number of qualified members" of its faculty to the hospital staff.

Former Rush faculty members were to be designated "Rush Professors"—"to provide continuity between the old and the new organizations." Rush veterans understood this to cover not only Rush staff at the time of the agreement but also those who joined Presbyterian (and the university faculty) later.

But university administrators did not agree, and when papers came into their offices describing newcomers as "Rush," they crossed out the "Rush" part. In any event the nomenclature was honorific and apparently a nod to the feelings of those recently bereaved of their medical college. At the university it denoted neither special standing nor automatic professorship.

The University of Illinois, then a shadow of what it would become, was Presbyterian's second choice for affiliation. The hospital had tried Northwestern first—the city's other strong medical school. But Northwestern had just completed its affiliation with Wesley Hospital and was not ready for another.

First choice or not, the Illinois affiliation provided university appointments for the hospital faculty and made it easier to recruit house staff. At least half of these would eventually come from the University of Illinois. It also helped the hospital when it sought research grants.

University of Illinois students began coming immediately to Presbyterian. William Grove, later to spend his career at the university, much of it as dean of the medical school, was one of them. A senior student in medical school in 1942, he took classes at Presbyterian and was one of the first University of Illinois students to take a clerkship (do third- and fourth-year clinical studies) at Presbyterian.

For the most part, the university-hospital relationship went smoothly, in spite of what Dr. Grove later called an "uneasy" relationship among administrators. The uneasiness was there from the beginning, however more obvious it became later. But among medical staff and faculty there was generally cooperation, even comradeship.

Meanwhile, the war veterans returned beginning in 1946, greeted with a half-serious "Welcome back but not here" from some colleagues who saw increased competition for patients. Attending physicians had to start their practices over again. Surgeons who had not gotten board certification found places saved for them by Dr. Vernon David. One of these, Dr. Frederic de Peyster, joined David and Dr. R. Kennedy Gilchrist for practice in general surgery.

Once back on the West Side, de Peyster, one of Rush's most recent graduates, "picked up the ball to carry Rush into the future," as Bill Grove saw it at the time, assuming the role of a "quiet but key leader" in maintaining alumni interest and keeping quiet pressure up for some sort of Rush revival.

St. Luke's a few miles away was at a high point academically, what with University of Illinois appointments in orthopedics, plastic surgery, neurosurgery and the like. But these all dated from the thirties, which were a golden age for that institution (as the twenties had been for Rush Medical College). There had been no new appointments in 10 years. So there was a 10-year gap in age of the staff, not to mention a modicum of hard feeling about those who hadn't gone to war.

The house staff was older than had been normal. Some who had run field hospitals were reduced to interns when they returned. Most were married (the old rules had forbidden marrying during internship), but were expected to be on call 24 hours. During his internship months in the urology department, Dr. Philip N. Jones was not even allowed out of the hospital. In the department of medicine, it was two nights on, one off, two weekends on, one off.

Presbyterian was to have its postwar revival, but at St. Luke's disadvantages began to predominate. St. Luke's had patients, a solid reputation and a thriving Northwestern University clerkship (without full affiliation).

But it was off the beaten path, while Presbyterian sat alongside the route of the new Congress (later Eisenhower) Expressway, which was to be fully operative in 1960. Presbyterian thus was to be near a gateway to downtown from three directions. Northwestern had the same advantage north of the river. St. Luke's on the other hand, enjoyed no such visibility and accessibility, and its neighborhood was in sharp socioeconomic decline.

So was Presbyterian's, but again location made the difference. Presbyterian was in the world's biggest medical district, while St. Luke's was isolated. St. Luke's began to slip in recruitment of patients, doctors and employees.

Neither had St. Luke's suffered the trauma of disaffiliation from a major university, as had Presbyterian, which now, like a man or woman after a divorce, had to pull itself together. It was nothing like that at St. Luke's, where business continued pretty much as usual.

Neither did St. Luke's have money sources comparable to Presbyterian's. The Bevan and Sprague funds, for example, though not university-size, nonetheless were important for funding research and professorships. War's end was a peak time for St. Luke's. The slide was coming.

For Presbyterian it was another story. The immediate postwar period was a slough for Presbyterian. Full of "prominent, nationally known senescent doctors," as one Presbyterian veteran said, it was on the verge of either something great or something very bad. Staff had to be strengthened, weakened as it was by lack of new blood during the war, not to mention the University of Chicago split.

The board felt the same way. "The only way to make this a distinguished hospital," said trustee A. B. Dick, Jr., "is to get distinguished physicians." Presbyterian had some already. Dick wanted more. So did Alfred Carton, another board veteran, the lawyer for the hospital who had functioned as its part-time president in the thirties.

Management consultants Booz, Allen & Hamilton were called in—a move unheard of for hospitals at the time. Some eminent professor might have been consulted, but not a commercial, nonmedical consulting firm. Booz, Allen recommended funding full-time professors. Rush (Presbyterian) was supposed to be a postgraduate school. Let it be one then.

Most teaching hospitals worth their salt had full-timers. But Presbyterian's teachers supported themselves with their practices and taught interns and residents in their spare time. This worked with James Herrick and his contemporaries, but Herrick could function with little more than a microscope. Things had changed with the coming of the modern laboratory. World War II had started a revolution in academic medicine. Get salaried people, said Booz, Allen.

The first of these were Dr. George M. Hass, a pathologist, and Dr. Douglas A. McFadyen, a biochemist, who arrived in January of 1946. Hass, now professor emeritus at Rush-Presbyterian-St. Luke's Medical Center, was to exert national influence, training a dozen or more pathologists who later headed departments around the country. A great believer in basic research, he recorded gains in seeking out the causes of arteriosclerosis.

Two years later, in January of 1948, Dr. S. Howard Armstrong, Jr., came as Presbyterian's first full-time chairman of medicine. These were the nucleus of the new staff. Armstrong stood out among them as a colorful, dynamic leader, but neither he nor McFadyen were to remain.

Staff veterans welcomed the developments, determined as they were that Rush should one day reopen. Even before the 13th General Hospital had gone overseas, its members had recommended hiring new people. The hirings represented an important move by the board toward keeping alive hopes for a revived Rush Medical College. The University of Illinois relationship, cordial and valuable as it was, could be no substitute for a new Rush risen from its limbo state. The board had funds which it was expected to put to just such a use.

More would be needed, however. In April of 1950, A. B. Dick, Jr., was announced as chairman of a campaign to raise $5.5 million. It was the first general public subscription campaign in Presbyterian Hospital history. Philanthropic muscles were beginning to ripple.

In December of 1951, a full-time surgeon arrived, Dr. Edward (Ted) Beattie, from George Washington University medical school, in Washington, D.C. Beattie was to become, in September of 1954, Presbyterian's first full-time head of surgery.

Beattie and Dr. Fred de Peyster had known each other as interns at Peter Bent Brigham Hospital in Boston before the war. When de Peyster heard Presbyterian was looking for a chest surgeon, he told Dr. Edwin Miller, Presbyterian's head of surgery, about him. Beattie, then at Brigham, couldn't come to Chicago right away but came after a stint at George Washington.

When Beattie did come, he was greeted on his first two visits in Chicago fashion—once when a hospital security guard and doorman known as "Bill the cop" shot to stop a purse snatcher right in front of Presbyterian and again when there was a robbery on the floor of the Drake Hotel, where he and his wife were staying.

Surgical research began under Beattie; he generally revitalized the program in surgery. Once or twice when he was chairman, for instance, his staff read more papers at the Forum of Fundamental Sciences (part of the annual meeting of the American College of Surgeons) than the surgical staff of the much bigger University of Illinois medical school.

Beattie left in July of 1965 for Sloan-Kettering Institute in New York City, where he became medical director and head of general and thoracic surgery. He was succeeded by Ormand Julian, another full-timer, who was succeeded by Dr. Harry Southwick, a private practitioner.

Meanwhile, in September of 1950, progress was reported by

Presbyterian researchers in another field, cardiovascular medicine—specifically in the search for causes of arteriosclerosis. This was James A. Campbell's work. Campbell had arrived in March of 1949 as the fourth of the full-timers, the second in medicine, recruited by Armstrong, who had known him at Harvard, as director of the new cardiovascular research laboratory. A mere 31 years old, he was destined to spend his life at Presbyterian and was to become the second founder of Rush Medical College.

In some respects Campbell was an unlikely candidate for the honor. The oldest of three children of a Presbyterian minister in Rochelle, Illinois, 75 miles west of Chicago, he grew up poor but educated. He attended Knox College (class of 1939), a small liberal arts school in Western Illinois, on a scholarship.

Then he passed up a scholarship to the Yale University School of Drama because his father blocked the move, though the Broadway producer Brock Pemberton reportedly had guaranteed the young man parts in his plays. (These later included the immensely successful "Harvey," in 1944.) Campbell went instead to The University of Chicago medical school. There is probably no one who knew the outgoing, dramatic Campbell in later life who would doubt that he once considered the stage for a career.

After two years at Chicago, 1939 to 1941, he interrupted medical school to spend a year working in the university's pathology laboratory. Then he was off to Harvard Medical School, where he got his M.D. in 1943. While at Cambridge, he met and married a young Brookline, Massachusetts, school teacher and recent graduate of Boston's Wheelock College, Elda Crichton, from Johnstown, Pennsylvania.

He interned at the Harvard Service in Boston City Hospital, then worked for a year at that hospital's Thorndike Laboratory. In 1946 he entered the Army at Edgewood (Maryland) Arsenal, where he became something of an expert on mustard gas. In 1947 he took the Harvey Cushing fellowship in cardiac medicine at Johns Hopkins University Medical School, working on cardiac catheterization under Dr. Richard Bing. In 1948 Armstrong recruited him for Presbyterian.

At Presbyterian, Campbell set up the cardiac catheterization lab in the department of medicine, equipping it like a surgical room over the objections of the head of surgery, Dr. Vernon David. It was in this room that Campbell performed Chicago's first heart catheterization.

He and his family lived in Lake Forest. Their next-door neighbors, Cyrus and Mary Adams, were known to the Armstrongs. Cyrus Adams and Howard Armstrong's father had been friends at Princeton. Cyrus and Mary's daughter, Mary Adams Young, was the wife of George Young, a lawyer soon to be a trustee of St. Luke's Hospital. Mary Young and Elda Campbell became good friends, and so did their husbands. The friendship would prove extremely important to Presbyterian and St. Luke's hospitals.

The James Campbell–Howard Armstrong relationship unravelled, however. The two disagreed philosophically on the role of publicly funded medical institutions, for one thing. Indeed, Armstrong was to leave Presbyterian eventually for Cook County Hospital, which he believed in and which Campbell didn't. A gap yawned between the two, whatever the cause.

In any event, for reasons that are not clear and not clearly related to any disagreement he had with Armstrong, Jim Campbell walked away from Presbyterian less than three years after he arrived, leaving to be dean of the Medical School of Albany, New York, a part of Union College in Schenectady.

Off to Albany he went, young and young-looking. His first day on the job, he was taken for a student and told not to park in the staff parking lot. The incident was symbolic. Albany was a mistake, he later told a colleague, without saying why. Two years after he arrived there, when Armstrong was in the process of leaving Presbyterian, Dr. Edwin Irons, son of the former Rush dean, came out to Albany with an offer from a search committee. Campbell jumped at it and hurried back to become Presbyterian Hospital's second full-time chairman of medicine. He was a few months short of his 36th birthday.

At Presbyterian he instituted the weekly medical grand rounds, which became the best attended exercise in the curriculum. He presided, quizzing interns and residents about patients' treatment. The sessions were full of tension, humor and knowledge for some, but full of trouble for others. A lot of students were scared to death of Jim Campbell.

To a contemporary who had known him at Harvard, it was vintage Campbell, a mixture of the fascinatingly brilliant and the fascinatingly vindictive. Aggressive, vitriolic, a born debater, he used the grand rounds to weed out the mediocre and to educate the rest. Coming to what was essentially a community hospital with 350 to 400 beds, he found people he wanted to keep and others he didn't and moved accordingly to shape his staff.

Patients were sometimes amused by the experience, including friends of trustees. Wheeled from their rooms down to the A. B. Dick auditorium in the East (now Kellogg) Pavilion, they would listen while Campbell asked opinions from assembled "youngsters" (interns, etc.), pleased to be the object of so much attention.

But they weren't at the receiving end. One or two surgeons were "not very good," and Campbell "went after them all the time," the same contemporary said. Jim Campbell was not about to suffer fools gladly. He was hard on administrators too. He is said to have "driven out" the first he worked under, made it tough on the next one, who didn't last long, and forced the board to a choice between him and the third. Recollections differ, but a prominent trustee is among those who concede it's possible things happened that way.

Furthermore, he clashed with his nominal superior at the University of Illinois medical school, Dr. Harry Dowling, the chief of medicine. A full-timer like Campbell and like him a debater and persuader, Dowling often won the university faculty to his views.

Conflict was to some extent inevitable. Campbell had the manner and goals of an entrepreneur. Ambitious and impatient, he was also a "medical politician" who elicited "unbelievable support" from the hospital board, in the words of a Presbyterian old-timer.

Campbell began hiring other full-timers immediately, using

Presbyterian's strong financial base to improve its teaching and research capabilities. The first, in 1953, were Graettinger and Kark, followed in 1954 by Trobaugh.

Dr. John Graettinger, also from Harvard, joined Campbell in medicine and worked with him in the newly reestablished cardiovascular lab, which he later headed. Dr. Robert Kark, who held the Licentiate of the Royal College of Physicians of London and had also trained in the Harvard Service in Boston, was internationally known for his treatment of renal (kidney and kidney-related) diseases. He introduced renal biopsies, a powerful diagnostic tool, into the cardiovascular lab.

Dr. Frank Trobaugh, a classmate of Campbell's at Harvard, came to head hematology (the study of blood and blood-related diseases). Trained in pathology, he had headed the laboratories for U.S. forces in Europe during the war before returning to Harvard in internal medicine. At Presbyterian he set up laboratories for analyzing patient's blood, urine, and the rest. These labs were moved into Campbell's department of medicine.

Campbell and Graettinger were joined in March of 1954 by Dr. Joseph Muenster, who came as Presbyterian's first research fellow. He was just out of the Air Force, from St. Louis, and came on a two-year assignment. He was to stay for considerably longer than that, however.

As a sort of fringe benefit, Campbell told Muenster when he hired him that he would introduce him to James Herrick, the 94-year-old founder of cardiology. But the day before Muenster was to meet the great man, Herrick died. Herrick's death came fittingly, perhaps, at about the time Campbell and his colleagues were developing heart catheterization at Presbyterian, the landmark diagnostic technique for the disease Herrick had first described which replaced the electrocardiograph, which Herrick had first used to map the disease's progress.

A year later, Campbell hired another full-timer, this time in endocrinology, Dr. Theodore Schwartz. Schwartz came from Johns Hopkins University by way of Duke University, where since 1948 he had been studying under Dr. Frank Engel. Schwartz had taught Engel internal medicine while Engel taught him experimental endocrinology, and the two had taken their board examinations at the same time.

Schwartz arrived with his family in the summer of 1954 and stayed at the Campbells' Walton Street apartment on the city's Near North Side until he and his wife found a house in Evanston. The Campbells were vacationing at the time.

Campbell had set up the endocrinology section which Schwartz headed with a Hartford Foundation grant. Other grant money followed, as one a few years later from the National Institutes of Health, to train cardiologists. Most of Presbyterian's grants came to the department of medicine.

Now there were five full-time salaried staff—the surgeon Beattie and medical men Campbell, Graettinger, Trobaugh and Schwartz—with Muenster as a fellow. An older physician who worked with this new team was Dr. Richard B. Capps, who also had served in the Harvard unit at Boston City Hospital. Capps was internationally known for his work in liver diseases.

Another, a part-timer, was Dr. Samuel G. Taylor III, who moved out of endocrinology to make room for Schwartz and went into oncology (the study of tumors). Taylor became the founder of oncology at Presbyterian.

Not all supported the changes. Some practitioners, volunteer teachers suspicious of this new breed of salaried full-time professors, called them "hired hands." But for these critics the worst was yet to come, as Campbell made changes in house-staff education and even in the hospital wearing apparel of attending physicians.

Meanwhile, "cutting-edge" diagnostic procedures were becoming available. Chief among them was cardiac catheterization, a much more powerful tool than the electrocardiograph, which up to then was the best available in Chicago. Heart surgery developed in tandem with the new diagnostic procedure. Cardiologists identified problems, and surgeons solved them.

Graettinger and Muenster supervised postoperative management when necessary. In this they worked closely with Beattie, who as chairman of surgery was Campbell's surgical counterpart, and the 20-year Presbyterian veteran, Dr. Egbert Fell. In 1956 Fell performed Chicago's first successful open-heart operation in which the heart-lung machine was used. This was at Cook County Hospital; a week later he did the second at Presbyterian Hospital. In 1957 he reported on his successful series of such operations (about 25) to the Chicago Surgical Society. The hospital's fame spread.

Campbell had left lab work in Graettinger's and Muenster's hands and had turned to administration and the training of house staff. Presbyterian's training programs were in need of improvement. In August of 1954, when Graettinger arrived, the hospital had only four interns.

A recruiting program was started, and the numbers of interns and residents grew rapidly. One year, seven residents came from Harvard Medical School. Clerkships for third-and fourth-year undergraduate clinical students also increased. University of Illinois students began to ask for Presbyterian for their third and fourth years. In time, well over half of University of Illinois clerks were being trained at Presbyterian.

During this time, not all the initiative was Campbell's. Members of the research and education committee met in 1955 to discuss how to spend a $25,000 Sprague Institute grant. The group included Ernest Irons, the former Rush dean; veteran surgeons Vernon David and R. K. Gilchrist, and Dr. Karl Klicka, the hospital's superintendent, whom Campbell opposed. It didn't include Campbell.

Campbell continued to attend to hospital-wide concerns, among which he considered none more important than providing a single standard of care for patients.

In Boston he had seen the best of the dual system—separate treatment for paying and nonpaying patients. His and Graettinger's chief at Massachusetts General Hospital, Dr. William B. Castle, knew his patients by name and came to see them at all hours, not just in the daytime. Nonetheless these patients, captive in their poverty, were used by doctors for clinical investigation.

When this happened under doctors like Castle, it was the reason American medicine developed rapidly between the wars. Doctors did this sort of clinical research (and teaching) in places like Cook County Hospital or Presbyterian's "lower wards," as they were called.

The private-patient pavilions, on the other hand—Phillips House at Massachusetts General in Boston, Harkness at Presbyterian in New York City, Passavant in Chicago and others —were regarded by medical students as "dogs," because in these places students had to stand and watch while the attending physicians did the work. They much preferred public institutions, where they could do it themselves and learn to be doctors.

Campbell decided this had to change. The double standard had to go because of what it meant to medical trainees (clerks, interns, residents) and paying patients as well as to nonpaying ones.

In the old system, trainees dealt mostly with more severe problems which were harder to treat outside a hospital and with patients who, because of their poverty, were relatively inert consumers of health care. The patients couldn't talk back because they had no choice. Thus the nature of ailments treated and the relative lack of questioning by patients prepared the trainees for only one kind of service.

Paying patients, on the other hand, were denied the improved care that stems from inquiry by trainees, who approached problems with a fresh eye. Every student remembers the day he caught something important that others had missed, Dr. John Graettinger observed. The atmosphere of inquiry meant better care for the paying patient.

Thus all patients became teaching patients, to be assigned to students and studied by house staff, and nonpaying patients were to have senior attending doctors assigned to them. Paying patients objected almost not at all. Instead, they welcomed the attentions of the eager, inquiring young learners. The learners relished the experience.

Private and nonpaying patients were roomed together, rather than the former in the private pavilion and the latter in the big open wards of the Murdock Building.

It was one of Campbell's most important contributions. In achieving it he was far ahead of developments that were to attend the coming of Medicare and Medicaid in the sixties, when many nonpaying patients became paying patients. Presbyterian Hospital became a superb example of how a single-standard system could work.

Meanwhile, Campbell made another move that affected medical education, a power play that worked. It had to do with deployment of interns and residents who traditionally were assigned to attending physicians—master doctors to whom they were apprenticed.

Instead, in 1957 as chief of medicine, Campbell assigned them "geographically" to wards, where patients themselves were assigned according to illness or injury. This was good for the patients, who became more accessible to their interns and residents, and it was good for the interns and residents, who no longer had to follow the master doctors on their appointed rounds.

But whether good or not for attending physicians, they did not appreciate the change. Some were used to being met at the hospital door by intern or resident, who helped them off with their coats, ran errands and otherwise made themselves useful. If the young men were late, the senior doctor would sometimes stand in the lobby, watch in hand, waiting.

The change did not affect surgery, centered as it is in the operating room. But it represented a dramatic shift of power from the private-practitioner, volunteer faculty to the academician. While the old way flattered the master doctor—"the chief" of his own "service"—the new way tended to deflate him.

Boston, Baltimore and New York City had made this change. But in Chicago and Philadelphia, two major centers, the best of the old died last. The system which had placed a student doctor at the feet of a Herrick, Woodyatt or Sippy gave way to one in which the young men became "house staff," still learning in a "service" but no longer tied to one teacher. The new system also provided for more give and take between teacher and student, and accepting things on the senior doctor's authority became less common.

There were objections, but Campbell won out. He was in charge and acted with the support of the trustees, who may not have fully understood the changes but trusted Campbell.

Campbell then introduced a physician's uniform, the white coat already worn by the salaried "hired help." Some of the private practitioners called it a "butcher's apron," but now they would have to wear one while in the hospital. Accustomed to dressing as their affluent patients dressed, they got used to dressing like the full-timers. Again Campbell had to fight to get his way, but he did it adroitly, and in the end this change was also accepted.

He had not run out of ideas, however. When some years later as president he had a Professional Building put up for practitioners' offices, some of the practitioners again drew the line. Nobody in his right mind will abandon the Loop, they argued. Their Michigan Avenue patients would not come to the West Side. But again Campbell prevailed: the Professional Building went up, and eventually almost the entire staff officed in it.

Campbell did none of this in a historical vacuum. The unused Rush charter was still alive. The Presbyterian laboratories, built in times past by people who in some ways thought like Campbell, were much in use. Presbyterian had been a major teaching hospital of a major university with its own commitment to research. When Campbell had come with his plans— one might say his grand plan—he found an institution groaning to be reborn. He didn't invent the atmosphere of inquiry, but he certainly built on it.

Though not yet chief executive, Campbell was developing the hospital along medical school lines, and people were beginning to notice. He enlarged the department of medicine, which he headed, using what money there was to pay competent "cronies" to head subsections and specialties. Some of the sections and subsections, like cardiology, did well, while others did not. He started the concept of fellowships at Presbyterian.

A fervent promoter of the private sector, he himself never practiced privately. Indeed, for a time he looked down on doctors who took money from patients. He retreated from this attitude a few years later, when as president he came to respect the practitioner's role. But he never wavered in his belief in salaried people, whom he considered necessary for overseeing the education of interns, residents and fellows.

He was also largely responsible for the hospital's decision at this time to stay in the city—when suburban migration was appealing to many a business and institution.

Campbell during these years was a free-wheeling type who thrived on directness, even bluntness. When his new endocrinologist, Ted Schwartz, was investigated by a federal officer, Campbell yelled out of his office to Schwartz asking him if he were a communist. "Some guy here wants to know," he hollered. Schwartz had refused to fire a technician who was suspected of communist tendencies.

When a senior physician complained about Schwartz's questioning of a patient during grand rounds, Campbell immediately called Schwartz in so the man could complain to his face. The accuser became flustered, and the matter was dropped.

When Schwartz, new in town and lacking a personal physician, came to work one day with sharp abdominal pains, he told Campbell. They decided it was appendicitis, and Campbell thought it was funny. It was as if the fly had caught up with the elephant, this specialist falling prey to one of the most common of internal ailments.

Campbell was on a roll, and he knew it. He was having more fun than a long Broadway run would have given him had he taken up play-acting. And the best was yet to come.

The Merger & Campbell's Accession to the Presidency 1955–1965

When Jim Campbell moved back to Chicago in 1953, he resumed his regular, even daily, contact with George B. Young, who had become a St. Luke's Hospital trustee in the early fifties. Campbell found a kindred spirit in the young lawyer whose parents were Yale professors, his father of history, his mother of English. To Young, Campbell put his ideas about merging Presbyterian and St. Luke's hospitals. It was the first Young heard of it. In lawyer Young's view, Campbell "had a patent" on the idea.

The two discussed it between chess games at each other's house or apartment. The Youngs and Campbells lived at first in apartments on the city's Gold Coast, a high-rent district north of the river and east of Michigan Avenue. Later they moved to Lake Forest, where the Campbells built a house on 20 acres of land that Marshall Field III, also a St. Luke's trustee, had bought from the Ogden Armour estate. Both Young and Campbell had met Field at a party. Field had put Young to work for him. Eventually Young was to head Field Enterprises.

137

Campbell had a plan for the two hospitals that he had been turning over in his mind since even before the Albany assignment. Now he bent Young's ear with it night after night, pushing the notion that neither hospital by itself had the "critical mass" (enough staff and facilities) to make the kind of institution he envisioned.

Another Presbyterian-St. Luke's connection was between St. Luke's trustee and later board president John P. Bent and his friend and Lake Forest neighbor, John M. Simpson, a Presbyterian trustee. On at least one occasion, a merger was discussed by Bent and Simpson.

St. Luke's at the time consisted of five buildings, including the aging five-story Smith Memorial at 1439 South Michigan Avenue and the 20-story high-rise built in the twenties at 1440 Indiana Avenue. In effect there were two hospitals that had to be connected by a third if they were to function as one. The third would be very costly. The huge wards of the Indiana Avenue building had already been divided to make more functional smaller wards or private rooms. The whole St. Luke's plant was crying for repairs and remodeling, all of which would have been expensive also.

Presbyterian, on the other hand, was expanding at a steady pace. Its new nursing school had gone up in 1952 at 1743 West Harrison. Its new East Pavilion was planned for six stories, with the option for seven more, on Congress Street opposite the new expressway. Both institutions faced continued costs which were to be met mostly by philanthropic donations. Comparable in size and serving comparable clienteles, they were to be competing for the same gift dollar.

The St. Luke's trustees discussed other merger possibilities —Northwestern and The University of Chicago—but contacted only Presbyterian. There was the feeling that the St. Luke's identity would be lost in a merger with one of the universities. St. Luke's might have continued on its own, in John Bent's opinion, raising the money for the needed connecting building. The institution wasn't as bad off financially as some claimed, though it did lack an endowment.

But if there were a merger, it was clear who would have to move. St. Luke's, run-down, needing a new building and isolated, would have to join Presbyterian in the soon to be booming Medical Center District on the West Side.

By October of 1955, both institutions were discussing merger. John Bent as St. Luke's board president explained the St. Luke's options to the press. It could stay where it was, repairing its buildings, or move to a university campus or merge with another hospital. Norman A. Brady, Presbyterian's assistant director, in a separate statement confirmed a report that discussions had been going on since the summer of 1954.

Discussions continued, obviously, and in a few months the decision was made. On February 10, 1956, the two boards voted to merge. On the St. Luke's side, where the move would be required, it was not an easy decision. The move was immensely unpopular with the medical staff, for one thing. "You couldn't blame them," said trustee George Young decades later, adding with a smile, "but we did blame them." The St. Luke's trustees voted two to one for merger, and then only after some "arm twisting" by the board's leaders.

The move would "combine two eminent groups of doctors who with a strong board (could) provide Chicago and the midwest with one of the country's foremost voluntary teaching hospitals," Ralph A. Bard, Sr., president of the Presbyterian board, and John Bent, the St. Luke's board president, told reporters. In addition, the Presbyterian connection would give St. Luke's a "direct" university affiliation (with the University of Illinois) and a new location which allowed room for expansion.

Two months later it was official. Bard was chairman of the new joint board, Bent its president. A $9-million fund drive was announced, to increase the new Pavilion "probably to 12 stories," thus adding 180 beds. It was time to say something like "Presbyterian and St. Luke's are dead. Long live Presbyterian-St. Luke's." But it didn't happen that way.

Bent had received letters and telegrams from staff members and trustees telling him not to do it. The woman's boards and nursing schools didn't like it a bit. For many it was an arranged marriage, "for the good of the children" (patients), as staff president Dr. Andrew Thomson told the medical staff 28 years later.

It was like merging U.S. Steel and Bethlehem Steel. The two groups were similar. They thought alike and had gone to the same or similar schools. Many of the doctors knew each other from the People's Gas Building, where Presbyterian and St. Luke's doctors had offices on the 14th floor. But they still didn't like it, and differences among them almost killed the merger.

It didn't help that Presbyterian had switched to the geographic system of assigning interns and residents (to wards), while St. Luke's still used the service-chief approach (assigning them to attending physicians), which better served the doctors' convenience.

Neither did the presence of full-time staff physicians at Presbyterian contribute to the St. Luke's staff's sense of well-being. These full-timers were the ones whom some called "hired help" and even treated as if they were. In the competition for department chairmanships, furthermore, the full-timers were automatic winners. Thus Campbell headed medicine, George Hass pathology, Ted Schwartz the endocrinology section, etc.

Some who lost out in competition for department chairs retired or left for other institutions—one to Northwestern and others to the University of Illinois or University of Chicago hospitals. For years after the merger, it was common to hear references to whether one was from Presbyterian or St. Luke's. Even patients got the message. Some asked to be placed in the "St. Luke's section," meaning the East (later Kellogg) Pavilion, newly built in time for the completed merger— rather than in Jones or other older Presbyterian buildings.

Milder reservations were registered by the genial and literate veteran St. Luke's surgeon, Geza De Takats, in *The New England Journal of Medicine* shortly after the physical merger. In the January 21, 1960, issue, De Takats applied Parkinson's Law to "the merging phenomenon": work expands to fill time available for its completion; subordinates multiply without increase in productivity. With institutions as with individuals, De Takats wrote with tongue in cheek, the more helpers and telephones one has, the more important one is. After the merger, "the money bag is full, and the administrator looks powerful." Yet to be learned, however, was "whether Mr. Jones, the man on the street, gets as much good service as he did in the premerged situation."

Resistance was diluted to a considerable degree through the medical staff presidency of Dr. George W. Stuppy, a University of Chicago and Presbyterian veteran, who edged the St. Luke's surgeon, Foster McMillan, in a 1956 election for the post. There was electioneering on both sides, but the choice was a good one.

Stuppy was an old hand at smoothing conflicts, partly because he had both the M.D. and Ph.D. and knew what it was to bridge hostile camps. He did a lot to smooth this conflict, among other things keeping it to himself when an overzealous St. Luke's trustee asked him to resign his newly won presidency.

A World War II 13th Hospital veteran who had served though over draft age, Stuppy had earlier helped form the Chicago Arthritis Club, later called the Chicago Rheumatism Society. After the war he headed an arthritis clinic at Presbyterian. He died in July of 1986.

The moment finally came, on June 26, 1959, when the doors of St. Luke's closed, 94 years after Reverend Clinton Locke and the members of Grace Episcopal Church had opened its doors in a small wooden house on State Street. The last patient, a Flossmoor woman, was given a corsage. Moving of patients had begun in February. The hospital had stopped admitting new patients on June 19th.

The five buildings were for sale. During the 1960 gubernatorial campaign, candidate Otto Kerner said the state ought to buy them. He won the election, but the state didn't buy them. A developer announced plans for converting them to a geriatric hospital. Various other uses were discussed and implemented over the years. In 1986 the two main buildings still stood.

The former Smith Memorial, five stories plus a penthouse at 1439 South Michigan Avenue, was empty and surrounded by vacant property. The 20-story building, erected in the 1920s at 1440 South Indiana Avenue, was a privately owned apartment building for the elderly and handicapped.

The St. Luke's Woman's Board had its last meeting in January of 1959, six months before the move. Its fashion show had been a joint venture with the Presbyterian Woman's Board for the three years since the legal merger. Emily Fentress Ott, the president of the newly combined Woman's Board, was the niece and namesake of Mrs. John W. Gary, president of the St. Luke's Woman's Board from 1926 to 1944. The following year's fashion show chairman was to be Mrs. Herbert C. DeYoung, who remains active on the board today.

The two woman's boards merged a few months later, though with some initial discomfort. The more church-oriented Presbyterian group had some adjustment to make when it began participating in the socially more high-powered St. Luke's activities. Like the doctors, however, both sides saw it through, and in years to come the Presbyterian-St. Luke's Woman's Board was to perform prodigious fund raising for the institution, in addition to a variety of service functions.

Among palpable benefits to the newly joined institution was the addition of St. Luke's surgeons to the staff mix. Joining the nationally renowned Beattie, who before and after the merger was most responsible for the institution's reputation for surgery, were Doctors Ormand Julian, Foster McMillan, Geza DeTakats, Eric Oldberg and others.

Julian, a national pioneer in cardiovascular surgery, promoted the use of a certain type of incision in open-heart surgery and performed the first successful resection and grafting for aneurism. DeTakats, one of the founders of vascular surgery, was an authority on the role of the sympathetic nervous system in vascular disease.

They joined Dr. Egbert Fell, a veteran Presbyterian surgeon who successfully performed heart surgery before the advent of the pump, or heart-lung machine, and was the first in Chicago to do so with it. Julian also performed pre-pump surgery, though after Fell.

Julian succeeded Beattie as head of Presbyterian-St. Luke's Hospital's department of surgery in January of 1966. Later, Dr. William Hejna headed surgery as an associate dean (not chief of surgery as before) of Rush Medical College in the early seventies. Dr. Penfield Faber succeeded Hejna in this post when Hejna became dean.

Another of the St. Luke's surgeons was Dr. Eric Oldberg, who in 1960 was to become president of the Chicago Board of Health—a position he held until 1979. Oldberg, considered a founder of neurosurgery in Chicago—with Dr. Percival Bailey of The University of Chicago, Dr. Loyal Davis of Northwestern and Dr. Adrien Verbrugghen of Presbyterian Hospital—headed that specialty at the University of Illinois in the thirties as he did at St. Luke's and at the new Presbyterian-St. Luke's. Oldberg died in June of 1986 at 84 after a distinguished civic as well as professional career.

Nursing was another problem area during the merger. It was another case of two rich traditions trying to meld, with powerful loyalties colliding—not the easiest of tasks. Symbols naturally meant much, as they do in any society. Thus such a thing as the nurse's cap became a matter of negotiation and even tension.

The two nursing schools were worthy of each other. Presbyterian's in the late forties had multiplied college and university affiliations and added psychiatry and tuberculosis work to its disciplines. In 1952 the Presbyterian school got a new Sprague building, at 1743 West Harrison Street, replacing the old Sprague home on Congress Parkway, torn down to make room for the new expressway. This 300-room, 14-story structure was renamed Schweppe-Sprague in 1960 to reflect both Presbyterian and St. Luke's origins. The Schweppe School for Nurses was part of the St. Luke's complex built in the forties.

The master of the merger by all accounts was Dr. James Campbell. But its mistress was Edith Payne, who managed the nursing side of the union. Payne had come to St. Luke's as director of nursing education in June of 1953 from Philadelphia Woman's Hospital. She succeeded the retiring Madeleine McConnell, who had held the position since 1939. Payne was the first St. Luke's nurse with a master's degree. Hers was from Columbia University. She valued nursing research, that is, the systematic observation and evaluation of how nurses performed their daily tasks.

To this end she hired a nurse researcher and began an overhaul of St. Luke's training and practice. At weekly meetings with her faculty, she tried to make training coincide with practice. She began a program of getting her faculty back to school.

In September of 1956, Payne was put in charge of the school of nursing at the newly merging institution. She moved immediately to Presbyterian, where she was joined shortly by nurses Barbara Schmidt and Dorothy Jane Heidenreich and researcher Josephine Jones. They began at Presbyterian the methods improvement work they had been doing at St. Luke's.

Schmidt and Heidenreich, who had been developing a policy and procedures manual for St. Luke's, were given a new task at Presbyterian, where they evaluated the system in use on the newly remodeled second floor of the Jones Building. The changes they recommended for "two Jones" were followed.

Strengthening the St. Luke's group's hand at Presbyterian was the presence of Norman A. Brady, hospital administrator under Dr. Karl Klicka, the superintendent. Brady had done an administrative residency at St. Luke's and helped in work-simplification efforts there. Now he worked again with Payne and her helpers, putting observers on the floors around the clock. From their reports he decided what changes were in order—installation of ward clerks to relieve nurses of clerical duties, for instance, and use of an automatic envelope-addressing system.

Brady also improved the central supply operation, relieving nurses of work such as sterilizing instruments and improving the system for getting drugs to the wards, so they arrived in patient-dose sizes rather than in big drums.

Payne was never rattled and found something to laugh about in inconvenient situations. For instance, she made do with various temporary offices while waiting for Sylvia Melby, her Presbyterian counterpart, to retire. One was the first-floor party room at Sprague, next to a serving kitchen. Even after

Melby's retirement, she officed for a time in the private-duty nurses' lounge of the new East Pavilion, during construction delays. Here she was joined now and then by a nurse who came to eat her lunch while the unflappable Payne worked at her desk.

Neither did Payne quail in the face of problems connected to the merger. To help this along, she set up joint committees and a nursing council which cleared changes in both institutions before the physical merger. Thus when the physical merger came, practices were alike in both places.

If one school had afternoon tea, the other got it. Presbyterian student government activities exceeded those at St. Luke's, so St. Luke's activities were strengthened. The alumnae associations were integrated. By the time of physical merger, the two institutions were very much alike.

Fund raising for the new institution was an immediate priority. The $9-million drive announced in April of 1956 was chaired by John Bent and insurance executive Donald R. McLennan, Jr. Mayor Richard J. Daley and his wife came to the kickoff dinner, where banker and trustee Philip R. Clarke was speaker.

The mayor also came for the laying of the Pavilion cornerstone in the spring of 1957, along with Bent, McLennan and a variety of clergy in ceremonial robes. The mayor had been in office less than two years at the time. His appreciation of the Presbyterian-St. Luke's venture was clear from the start, as was his political support.

The eight-story, 80-apartment Kidston residential building for house staff and their families had gone up in 1955. In 1959, the 56-room McCormick Apartments for nursing students was completed. Seven stories high, the building, named after Colonel Robert R. McCormick of the Chicago Tribune, was paid for in part by a $300,000 grant from the McCormick Foundation. This was in addition to rooms already available for nursing students in the Sprague (soon to be Schweppe-Sprague) School of Nursing Building.

The Jelke Memorial, a $3.5-million medical science research building, was opened in 1960. Oleomargarine maker

John F. Jelke gave $1 million to help build it. McCormick and Jelke were part of an $18.5-million expansion under way since 1956. The blueprint for this expansion was provided by management consultants Booz, Allen & Hamilton after a seven-month study.

Presbyterian-St. Luke's was hailed in news accounts as approaching Massachusetts General Hospital in Boston, John Hopkins University in Baltimore and Columbia-Presbyterian in New York City in size and services, with an expected patient capacity of over 1,000 beds—almost double the 554 it had in 1960. Jim Campbell's "critical mass" had been achieved.

The merger was the best thing that ever happened to the two medical staffs and a complete overall success, said critics and supporters of Campbell alike years later.

And by common agreement, it was Campbell's doing. He gave the merger direction, working hard and insisting on excellence, though making enemies along the way. He gained support for it from board and staff. He put the whole thing through. It was a triumph of personal diplomacy achieved by playing largely behind the scenes. That was about to change.

The merger orchestrated, full-timers in place, geographic placement of house staff achieved, James A. Campbell stood in the late fifties as a first among equals at Presbyterian-St. Luke's, minister plenipotentiary without portfolio.

He had planted the seed of the merger idea and had seen it grow to harvest. The institution meanwhile was being run in what he considered an undistinguished manner. And he was not alone in his thinking.

Influential trustees like John P. Bent and A. B. Dick III found themselves looking askance at practices that to them were unbusinesslike. Staying in the black, to them an unquestioned imperative, was apparently only an attractive option to some administrators. The medical staff did little to oppose this view. Doctors sometimes proposed buying equipment, for instance, without due regard for its economic feasibility.

Indeed, those were simpler days, and hospital business was conducted in near hip-pocket fashion. Room rates would be raised on a show of hands by the medical staff at the University Club after a presentation by the hospital director.

The solution was to put a businessman in charge. Herbert Sedwick, a Commonwealth Edison retiree, became executive vice president in 1957, general manager in 1959, chairman of the executive committee in 1960 and life trustee and president in 1963 after two others had had short, unhappy terms as president of the merged institution.

Sedwick's dollars-and-cents approach was what the trustees, if not the doctors, ordered, though some of the latter came to endorse profitability too. He "put the organization on its feet," said one doctor. To John Bent he was "a pillar of strength" for the institution. One of his early moves, however —separating nursing education from nursing service—did not set well with some staff. It was a classic mistake to split the two, according to a close Campbell associate, and indeed Campbell later reversed the move.

Meanwhile, Campbell wanted the job. If he asked himself why he shouldn't have it—and there is no evidence he did—he would have come up with no good answers. Seated in the chair of medicine, he had already effected big changes. Seated in the presidency, he could do much more.

So he "maneuvered" and "shouldered" his way, as a colleague put it, building his base and staying close to the board. Sedwick stayed long enough to do his duty as he saw it and then asked out. Bent filled in, and a search was announced. George Young, by now chairman of the board, said the board wanted a president such as major academic institutions wanted, one who would be responsible for policy and planning and would report directly to the board, whose representative he would be. Reporting to this president would be an executive vice president, who would handle operations.

Young knew whom he wanted, if some trustees didn't. His business was to educate them to the merits of James A. Campbell, on the one hand, and to keep Campbell from bolting, on the other. New York's Mount Sinai Hospital, the University of Washington and the University of Arizona were institutions who shared Young's opinion about Campbell.

Offers were made. Arizona was ready to hire Graettinger, Trobaugh and Schwartz along with Campbell in a sort of medical-education power play. At one point, the three besides

Campbell were getting bulletins on the half hour about the progress of negotiations, which apparently were not successful.

The trustees presumably got wind of these near misses and possibilities, among which the Mount Sinai offer loomed big enough to precipitate a decision. The charade, if it was one, ended. Young apparently convinced the last of the doubters some 18 months after he'd described the man they were looking for. He and Bent, to whom Campbell had become "the obvious choice," drove over to the house of Bent's fellow Lake Forest resident and made him their offer.

Jim and Elda Campbell and two guests were at dinner. "Come with us," said Young to Campbell, who followed him and Bent into an adjoining room. Campbell, the next president of Presbyterian-St. Luke's Hospital, accepted on the spot.

Young announced it October 8, 1964. Campbell was to take office November 18. Norman A. Brady was to remain as executive vice president. In Campbell the institution had at its head a nationally known working physician-scientist, what in athletics might be called world-class performer.

He also was a businessman and a politician and "one of the toughest characters" Edward McCormick Blair, later to chair the board, ever met. A perfectionist, he came into office with tremendous imagination and big plans. His forceful approach was resented by some, his plans were questioned, but he is widely if not universally credited with achieving what he set out to do.

Essential to Campbell's success was the redefined presidency that came out of his first year in office. The president that George Young had described 18 months earlier was not a chief executive officer. He was rather a paid chairman of the board, or assistant chairman, who developed policy, got board approval for it, and interpreted it to the executive vice president, who headed operations.

The executive vice president was in effect the CEO. The EVP whom Campbell inherited, Norman A. Brady, was used to this arrangement. He naturally looked on Campbell as Mister Outside, dealing with the board and overseeing public relations and fund raising, and on himself as Mister Inside, running the hospital.

Nothing could have been further from the role Campbell had been carving out for himself. He was used to working with the board. But he was equally used to making things happen in the hospital. Nonetheless, he was not sure of the role he wanted to take as president, or so it appeared to Donald Oder, the Arthur Andersen partner who in August of 1965 undertook a study of the institution's corporate structure.

The financial executive was already reporting to Campbell, and the medical staff was going around Brady to do the same. The question was, did Campbell want to be chief executive officer? Oder, an old hand at servicing the hospital for Andersen, put the question to him, and Campbell decided, yes, he did want to be CEO.

In that case a second tier was called for, four vice presidents —one each for administration, finance, public relations and development, academic and medical affairs. Each would report to Campbell as president and CEO. Oder was promptly hired as vice president-finance. Brady became executive vice president-administration, keeping his title but not its full authority. Richard S. Slottow remained vice president–public relations and development. A few months later, Dr. Mark Lepper was made vice president–medical and academic affairs.

The structure remained in place into the mid-eighties, by which time it had become common in hospitals. But in 1966, when Oder came aboard, very few hospitals were so organized. A key element, in addition to putting Campbell in charge, was its combining medical and academic authority in one vice president, Lepper.

In this action a philosophical point was made in addition to a practical one, namely that patient care and teaching went together. Patient care personnel were teachers, and vice versa. The medical-school character of the institution, yet to be fully realized, served the hospital. There was to be education for the sake of patient care and research for the sake of education. Thus was organized the medical-academic institution that within a decade was to blossom as fruitful in its own right.

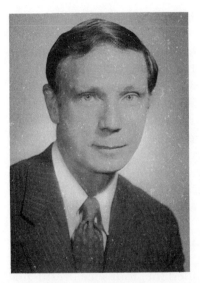

James A. Campbell, M.D.,
1917–1983.
(Photo by Fabian Bachrach)

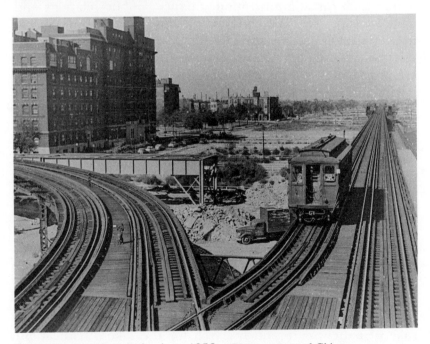

Presbyterian Hospital, circa 1953. *(Photo courtesy of Chicago Transit Authority)*

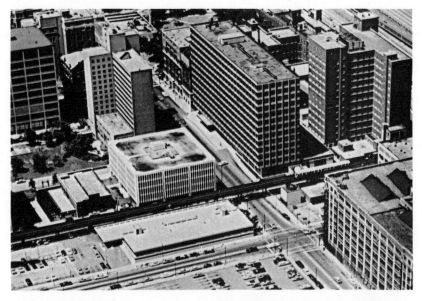

Aerial view of Presbyterian-St. Luke's Hospital in mid-1960s.

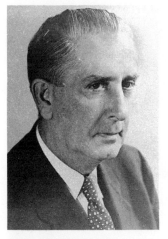

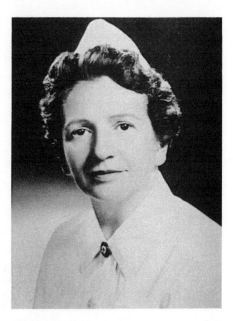

George W. Stuppy,
M.D., 1898–1986, first
president of combined
Presbyterian-St. Luke's
Hospital medical staff.

Edith D. Payne, R.N., 1903–1976.

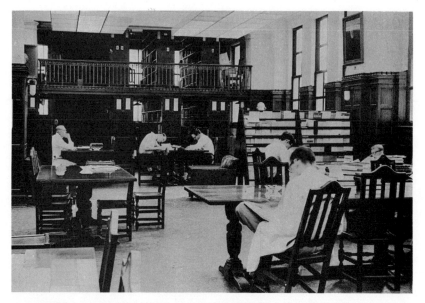

Rush Medical College library, mid-1960s.

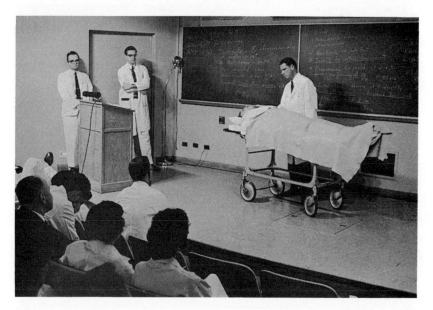

Grand Rounds, with James A. Campbell, M.D., presiding.

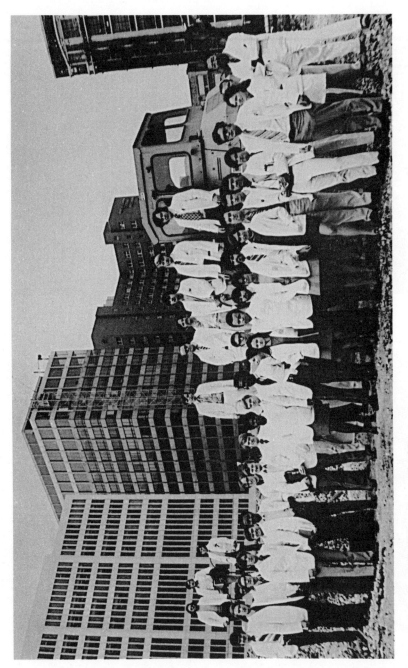

Rush Medical College class of 1974.

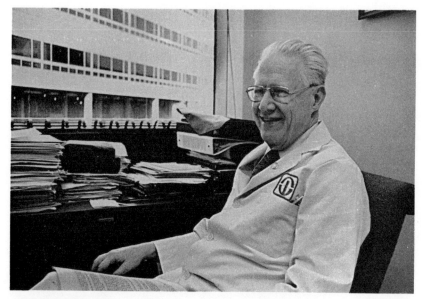

Mark H. Lepper, M.D.

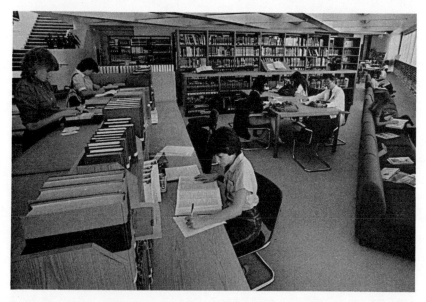

Library of Rush University.

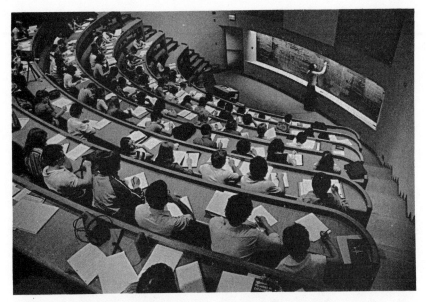

Lecture Hall of Rush University.

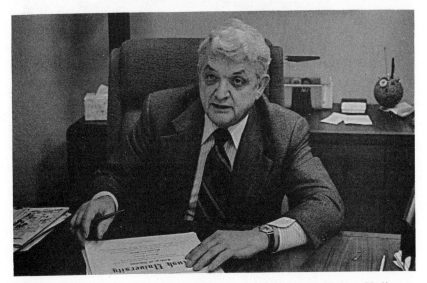

Luther P. Christman, R.N., Ph.D., the John and Helen Kellogg
Dean of the Rush University College of Nursing.

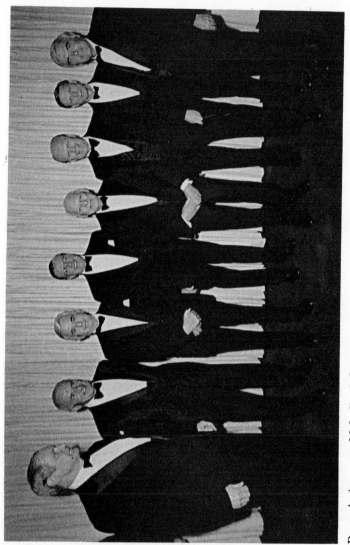

Past chairmen of Medical Center's Board of Trustees: (from left): George B. Young, John P. Bent, Edward McCormick Blair, Albert B. Dick III and Edward Blettner, with former President Gerald R. Ford, James A. Campbell, M.D. and Harold Byron Smith, Jr., chairman, in 1981.

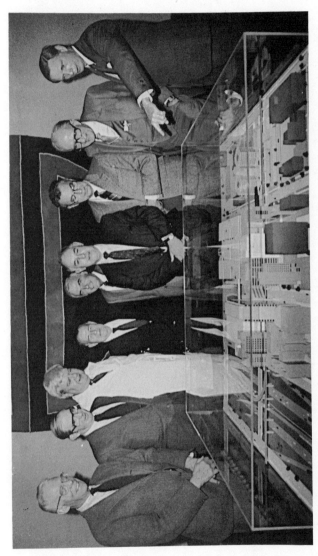

Past medical staff presidents in 1981 reviewed Medical Center development. (Left to right) Frederic A. de Peyster, M.D., Stanton A. Friedberg, M.D., Joseph J. Muenster, M.D., Trustee Frederick G. Jaicks, Trustee chairman Harold Byron Smith, Jr., Maurice L. Bogdonoff, M.D., Milton Weinberg, Jr., M.D., Robert J. Jensik, M.D., and James A. Campbell, M.D., president of Rush-Presbyterian-St. Luke's Medical Center.

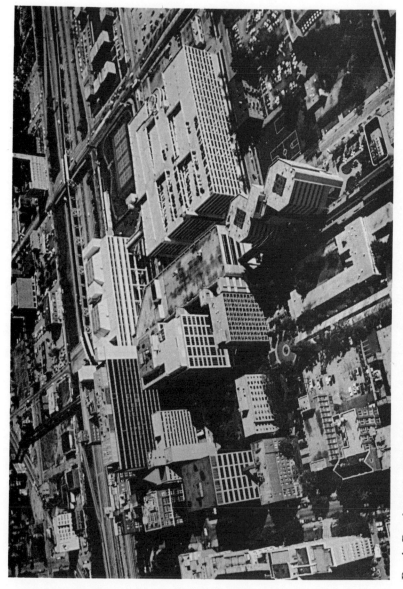

Rush-Presbyterian-St. Luke's Medical Center in 1983.

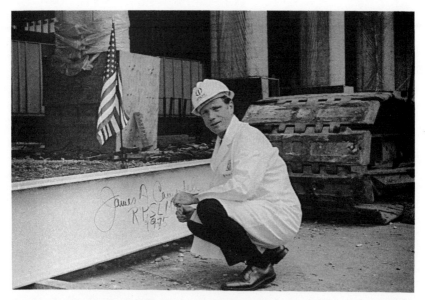

James A. Campbell, M.D., at "topping out" of Rush University
Academic Facility, 1975.

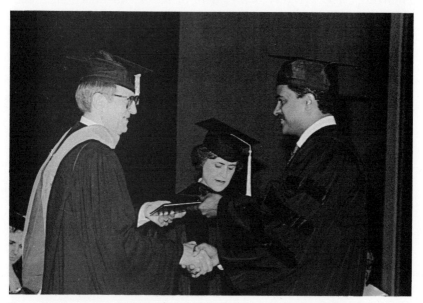

Donald R. Oder presided at 1984 Commencement exercises.

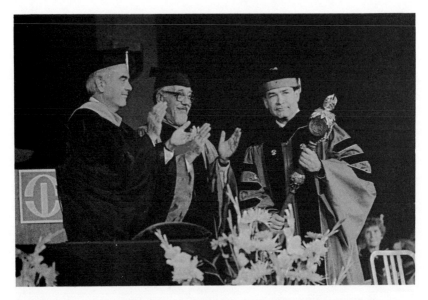

Harold Byron Smith, Jr., chairman of the Trustees, John S. Graettinger, M.D., university marshall, at installation of Leo M. Henikoff, M.D., (right) as president of Rush University, in 1985.

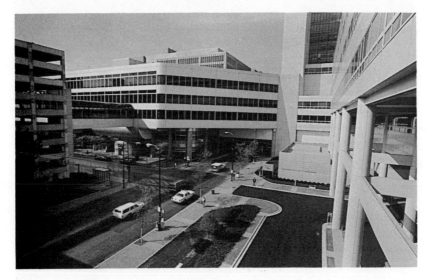

Rush University academic facility.

The Second Founding of
Rush Medical College
1963-1983

In March of 1963, trustees of Rush Medical College met with representatives of the American Medical Association to discuss how to make best use of Rush's assets. These totalled $1,677,000, including land and buildings then used by Presbyterian-St. Luke's Hospital. One of the options was to revive Rush.

Rush was a paper tiger. The school had gone out of business more than 20 years earlier. Its faculty had been appointed to the University of Illinois medical school, where they were known as "Rush professors." These teachers continued to teach third- and fourth-year medical students (clerks) at Presbyterian and later Presbyterian-St. Luke's Hospital. A few were careful also to preserve Rush as a legal entity.

Once or twice a year they met as trustees, often over lunch. With the help of retired investment banker and fellow trustee William J. Hagenah, they reviewed the endowment portfolio, never more than a half million dollars. Once a year they went through the motions, required by their charter, of appointing a Rush faculty, namely the staff of Presbyterian or Presby-

161

terian-St. Luke's Hospital. Thus the chairman of surgery at Presbyterian was not only a University of Illinois professor of surgery but a Rush professor as well. Through these and other activities, some of them formalities, the Rush charter was kept alive by a small group of loyalists.

The endowment income was put to use as well. For instance, half the salary of Dr. Friedrich Dienhardt, a virologist who with two other researchers, one of them his wife Jean, an immunologist, developed a new mumps vaccine, was paid by Rush for several years after his arrival at Presbyterian-St. Luke's in 1961. With Dr. A. William Holmes, the Dienhardt group also worked on cancer and hepatitis, experimenting on small, squirrel-like monkeys called marmosets.

The 1963 meeting with the AMA, therefore, was not an exercise in nostalgia. The Rush trustees, headed by their chairman, Dr. Frank B. Kelly, Sr., did not come to waste their time or that of the AMA man, Dr. W. S. Wiggins, secretary of the AMA's history-laden Council on Medical Education. In addition to Kelly, there were Rush trustees Dr. Frederic A. de Peyster, Dr. R. K. Gilchrist and Judge Hugo M. Friend and former trustee Charles L. Byron. They suggested three possibilities.

The Rush assets could be used to (a) start a new medical school or (b) enter on a more independent relationship with the University of Illinois or (c) set up a trust fund to aid medical education in general. A new school—of necessity a four-year, degree-granting institution—would cost $30 million to open and $3 million a year to operate for the first 10 years, Wiggins told them.

It was enough to stop the most dedicated in his tracks. The trustees didn't have the money to start a new school. If they wanted to revive Rush, they would have to find an umbrella university. They considered three possibilities: Illinois Institute of Technology, Roosevelt University and the University of Illinois. The last was an obvious choice, for reasons of proximity and familiarity.

A few weeks after the meeting with Wiggins, three Rush

trustees—Doctors Gilchrist, de Peyster and Fred O. Priest—presented the case for declaring Rush a second medical school of the University of Illinois to the dean of the university's medical school, Dr. Granville Bennett. Bennett said he was interested, but a few weeks later told de Peyster the outlook was not good.

The response smarted. Rush had the facilities, the teachers, even the students, that is, third- and fourth-year students (clerks) from University of Illinois and other medical schools. It had a history of "125 years [sic] of uninterrupted teaching," as Kelly reported to 35 or so Rush alumni a month later in Atlantic City.

The Rush alumni, members of an organization founded in 1868 and almost 3,000 strong, had a stake in reviving Rush. As one told de Peyster at the Atlantic City meeting, "This being a graduate of a defunct school is not good." Indeed it was not, and besides, the University of Illinois was getting "a tremendous bargain" from Presbyterian-St. Luke's, paying a mere $60,000 a year for the clinical education of one-third or more of its clerks.

"Pretty darn cheap" at the price, de Peyster commented at Atlantic City. Furthermore, the arrangement depended in part on use of the Rush-owned Senn and Rawson buildings, rented at a dollar a year by Presbyterian-St. Luke's hospital. "These are our buildings," de Peyster reminded the alumni.

And yet though university backing was necessary, University of Illinois backing (incorporation, actually) would place some uncomfortable limits on a revived Rush. For instance, all but five percent of its students would have to be Illinois residents. Eventually Rush was to accept just such a restriction when it accepted state funds given to educate Illinoisans who would practice in Illinois, but for now it was all talk.

Meanwhile, Rush trustees tended the flickering flame, nursed their modest funds and above all kept the charter from lapsing. Frank Kelly kept James Campbell, president of Presbyterian-St. Luke's from November of 1964, informed of his various meetings about the future of Rush. Campbell listened with interest but had to admit the time was not ripe for reviving Rush Medical College. It would soon be ripe, however, sooner than those hopeful Rush trustees and alumni dreamed.

The break came in 1967, when the Illinois Board of Higher Education asked Campbell to do a statewide study of medical education. He pulled together a staff for the project: Dr. Mark Lepper, Dr. W. Randolph Tucker and sociologist Irene Turner.

Their report issued the following year, "Education in the Health Field for the State of Illinois," or the Campbell Report, called for massive expansion of health profession education in Illinois and showed how expansion might be supported in public and private schools. Moreover, it convinced the legislature of the need and the funding solution. In the summer of 1969, the legislature voted to provide state aid for both private and public medical schools.

Even before this, the Rush ball had begun to roll. In November of 1967, the Rush trustees made what Campbell called a "statesmanlike and generous" offer to cede Rush Medical College to Presbyterian-St. Luke's Hospital with the understanding that the hospital would try to reactivate the college.

Hospital Trustee Chairman A. B. Dick III formed a committee headed by past chairman George Young to investigate the matter. On it were Chairman Dick, past Chairman John Bent, future chairmen Edward F. Blettner and Edward McCormick Blair, and trustees Elliott Donnelley and Arthur M. Wood. At the same time a national advisory council of top-rung medical educators was also convened by the trustees to consider the same question.

The stage was set for major developments. In 1968 the Campbell Report was issued. In July of that year the first of a series of meetings took place with University of Illinois representatives to discuss a new relationship with a reactivated, semi-independent Rush. The proposal was in effect what Rush trustees had wanted in 1963, namely a separate identity (Rush Medical College) within the university for "Rush professors" and Presbyterian-St. Luke's Hospital.

Negotiations went badly. Personalities and expectations clashed, communication floundered. Mutual respect was wanting. Rush wanted financial autonomy. Its people were not ready to submit to University of Illinois control, which they considered inadequate and ill-directed. The University of Illinois people were suspicious.

The university president, David D. Henry, told his people to work something out, and the university's medical faculty approved incorporation of Presbyterian-St. Luke's with a revived Rush Medical College as one of several university schools of medicine, each with its own dean under a university executive dean. Presbyterian-St. Luke's-Rush would become a "so-called semiautonomous" school, Campbell said. But it wasn't clear to either side what the other meant by "semi-autonomous."

Money was, not surprisingly, a major obstacle. Campbell wanted it from the state on a no-strings basis. But provost Lyle Lanier, the university's number two executive, drew the line there, saying that's not how state dollars were used. "There had to be accountability," Dr. William Grove, University of Illinois medical dean at the time, said years later.

But neither Campbell nor Lepper was willing to surrender the paymaster's role. They wanted to pay their own department heads with their own money. A compromise solution was offered by which Presbyterian-St. Luke's would have its own separate account from which to pay its department heads.

But more than a year went by without an agreement. George Young's committee and the national advisory group were at work nonetheless. By September, one issue at least was decided: Presbyterian-St. Luke's would merge with Rush to form a medical center that would include a revived Rush Medical College.

"We have a new opportunity to show that medical education belongs in the mainstream of medical care," Campbell told the hospital's medical staff on September 3, 1969, the day the hospital trustees voted to merge with Rush. On October 24, they signed the merger agreement, and Rush-Presbyterian-St. Luke's Medical Center became a legal entity.

There was still time for an agreement with the university, which was under pressure to double its output of doctors, but not much time. Rush Medical College would open in two years. For more than 70 years it had leaned on two major universities. Now there was no waiting on another institution.

A new proposal was made to the University of Illinois in November. This was turned down in January of 1970. In March the two institutions' 28-year connection was severed, effective the following March. "Go it alone," national advisory committee chairman Dr. Robert J. Glaser, acting president of Stanford University medical school, had advised the Presbyterian-St. Luke's trustees. And that's what they did.

Rush Medical College reopened on September 27, 1971, with 98 students—61 first-year (from 1,050 applicants), 31 third-year and six Ph.D. candidates. Rush became Illinois' seventh medical school and the nation's 108th. Yet it was not strictly a new school, and this qualified it for state and federal (matching) funds under "health manpower production" priorities.

As an existing school opening new positions for students, Rush qualified for state aid according to the formula spelled out in the Campbell Report and endorsed by the legislature. The other six medical schools also received aid as they opened new positions, but none of these were starting from scratch as Rush was, and none received as much.

Meanwhile, there was a changing of the guard among Rush Medical College trustees. Seven retired as trustees—Doctors Kelly, de Peyster, Gilchrist, Priest, Bertram G. Nelson and Robert Morse Potter and investment advisor William Hagenah. Other trustees of the inactive institution had retired in the sixties—Judge Hugo Friend after 26 years, Frederick C. Shafer, Earl Hostetter, Henry A. Gardner, Charles L. Byron, Dr. Vernon C. David, and Dr. Wilber E. Post. Four of the seven recent retirees—Kelly, Gilchrist, Potter and Hagenah —were elected by the medical staff to the Rush-Presbyterian-St. Luke's Medical Center board.

Rush opened with a three-year program, summers included,

which was not uncommon at the time; such was the urgency to produce doctors. Rush switched to the four-year schedule in 1973—a move defended by Dr. William Hejna, associate dean and later dean of Rush Medical College in *The Journal of the American Medical Association,* where he said the three-year program added few if any graduates, saved little or no money but made students more tired and otherwise less capable of pursuing their studies.

The Rush admissions process recognized competence in nonmedical fields and ignored some traditional requirements that were judged nonessential. Rush accepted more women and more older students than the University of Illinois, for instance. Ten percent of applicants were women, but 14 percent of those accepted were women—this without special effort to attract women students. The trend continued into the mid-eighties, when 35 percent of Rush students were women.

Some University of Illinois medical students transferred to Rush. The University of Illinois was in the midst of changes, and this process of transition didn't help the instructional situation. More important, thanks to Rush's partial subsidization in these early years by the state, there was no difference in tuition between the two institutions for Illinois residents. Besides, Presbyterian-St. Luke's clinical training for third- and fourth-year students (clerks) had been an attraction for decades.

A medicine clerkship at Presbyterian-St. Luke's, for instance, was considered a plum in the early seventies. So was the surgical clerkship, depending on the specialist one served under. Cardiac, oncologic and ear-nose-throat (ENT) surgery were special attractions. Some teachers stood out for their eagerness to help, such as Dr. Fred de Peyster and Dr. David L. Roseman, who seemed to welcome the chance to increase a student's knowledge.

Indeed, Presbyterian-St. Luke's Hospital had been almost but not quite a medical school. Half to two-thirds of University of Illinois third- and fourth-year students were trained there. Even so, Rush needed new structures—admissions and

registrar's offices, basic science departments, rules for govern-
ance, faculty contracts, and when the time came, a commencement ceremony.

Many basic science teachers were on hand—biochemistry
and pathology teachers, for instance. But physiology, anatomy
and other departments had to be established. Research space
was limited. Rush did not have an animal facility until 1976,
for instance. A separate research center was part of
Campbell's original plan, but it never materialized, notwithstanding Campbell's offer to the medical staff to put the name
on it of any doctor who put up the money for it.

These were growing pains in becoming a full-scale academic
medical center. Before these problems could be addressed,
however, there had to be a dean. Dr. Mark Lepper got the job
almost by default. In February of 1970, the search committee
told Lepper to contact Dr. Julius Richmond, of the State
University of New York at Syracuse, who was also deputy
director of Project Headstart in Washington, D. C. Lepper,
on his way to a Caribbean vacation, wrote Richmond a note
that through a series of mishaps was never mailed—and this
with the calendar counting and clock ticking to a projected
Fall, 1971 opening.

Lepper returned from his vacation some weeks later and
called Richmond, who of course knew nothing of the Rush
offer. Lepper told him the news, but Richmond had already
received an offer from Harvard Medical School which he
could not refuse. So Lepper, Campbell's right-hand man and
acknowledged resident philosopher, took the job. He held it
for three and a half years until the governor of Illinois tapped
him to head a state commission.

There were four associate deans, one for surgery, one for
medicine, one for biological and behavioral sciences, one for
student and faculty affairs. Dr. William F. Hejna, who later
succeeded Lepper as dean, was associate dean for surgical
sciences and services. Dr. Robert W. Carton held the same
post for medical sciences and services. Dr. Max E. Rafelson
held it for the sciences and Dr. John S. Graettinger for student
and faculty affairs. All four reported to Lepper, who as dean

oversaw not only medical education but also patient care—both medical school and hospital. Department heads reported to the associate deans, who were also assistant vice presidents. It was a structure that reflected the institution's joining of patient care and education.

Rush Medical College was a medical school organized for the benefit of a hospital, in the English manner. The hospital would remain no matter what happened to Rush. In it health professionals were educated in a patient-care, rather than a research, setting. Education served patient care, and research served education.

These were the three legs of the stool on which academic health centers were said to rest—patient care, education and research. Campbell argued for a fourth leg, management, to guarantee accountability and efficiency. Around this principle he organized his entire administrative structure and later, to this end, he promoted a master's program in health systems management at Rush University.

Closely linked to Campbell's emphasis on management was his emphasis on parity among health professions. He knew doctors would be "first among equals" in an academic health center, but he did what he could to save the rest from second-class status. Thus he made sure that deans of the College of Health Sciences and The Graduate College were made vice presidents and members of the management committee, as were their counterparts in medicine and nursing.

These were the dean of the college of medicine, who was vice president for medical affairs, and the dean of the college of nursing, who was vice president for nursing affairs. All four of these dual appointments evidenced the crucial symbiosis of practice with education.

Later deans of Rush Medical College included Dr. Leo M. Henikoff, who succeeded Dr. William Hejna in an acting capacity, and Dr. Robert S. Blacklow. Blacklow, who was dean from 1978 to 1980, is remembered for his keen interest in and enthusiasm for the college, including great support for the honor society, Alpha Omega Alpha. He also rewrote most of the bylaws for the college's alumni association, though not himself an alumnus. Blacklow's successor, Dr. Henry P. Russe, took office in February of 1981.

With Rush Medical College reactivated, a new academic health center begun and a senior health university in the offing, long-term planning was in order to produce facilities to house them. From the planning came three phases of facilities development. Phases I and II were primarily to start the new educational programs. Phase III was primarily to modernize patient care facilities. In each phase, however, there was overlapping.

Phase I involved adding two floors to the Jelke SouthCenter building for classroom space and six to the Professional Building; erecting a 1,500-car parking facility for visitors, patients and staff; and expanding various other parts of the medical and educational plant. It was completed in 1973 at a cost of $23.4 million.

In Phase II, the $24.5-million Rush University Academic Facility was built, and 883 parking spaces were added. The cost of the Academic Facility was covered by almost $15 million in federal and state money and $10 million in privately given and borrowed funds. Ground was broken for it in November of 1973; it was dedicated in September of 1976. Rush's longtime supporter and sometime patient, Mayor Richard J. Daley, helped with the groundbreaking, symbolically pushing a wheelbarrow, as the *Chicago Tribune* pictured him the next day on its front page.

Phase III, as we shall see, centered around a new nine-story patient-care facility connected to the rest of the complex.

The Academic Facility, built to house the colleges of medicine, nursing and health sciences, was the flagship structure of Rush University, which had been founded in 1972. Six stories high, with supports for six to eight more, it stretched down a narrow, busy strip of Paulina Street south of Harrison. Connected to the hospital over rapid transit "L" tracks, its concrete-block walls were partly filled with sand to block the noise of passing trains; its sealed joints were covered with sound-absorptive panels. The building had classrooms, laboratories, study areas and library, all linked by walkways or corridors to the hospital, Professional Building and Johnston R. Bowman Health Center for the Elderly.

The Bowman Center also opened in 1976, when there were very few "dyed in the wool geriatricians" in the U.S., according to its medical director, Dr. Rhoda Pomerantz. Dr. Pomerantz first came to Rush as a Presbyterian Hospital intern in 1962 and learned to look on the institution as "always one step ahead" of similar places.

In winning the Bowman Center contract, Rush competed successfully against seven other Chicago-area institutions, each of which proposed how to use a bequest by Lula Bowman, widow of dairy owner J. R. Bowman. Mrs. Bowman had designated the money for care of the elderly. The Northern Trust Company, as trustee of her estate, asked for ideas. The Rush proposal was to care for sick elderly patients with the goal of restoring them to relative self-sufficiency.

The 176-bed Bowman Center has its own board and independent legal existence but is managed by Rush. David W. Dangler, the Northern Trust officer who headed the search and became a Rush trustee after Bowman was established, chairs that board.

The building includes some residential apartments but is mostly for rehabilitation of its patients, who are gotten in and out as soon as is consistent with their health, always with a view to their returning home. After 10 years, in fact, three out of four Bowman Center patients were going home after treatment. The major challenge has been to give help at the right time to stroke victims and other similarly afflicted people so that fewer have to stay in nursing homes. In sum, Bowman is primarily for patients who can be restored to full or near-full social participation.

Rehabilitation is more than physical and involves counseling both patient and family, as regards use of community services such as "meals on wheels." A patient spends three months at the most at Bowman, up to twice as much for psychiatric rehabilitation as for medical. The Geriatric Assessment Program (GAP) involves evaluation of arrangements to be made for a patient and communication of the findings and rationale to the patient's family. Commitment to the patient extends past hospitalization, again with a view to de-institutionalizing of care.

Consistent with its commitment to geriatric work, Rush established an Alzheimer's Disease Clinical Center in 1985. Within two years, Rush had been designated one of Illinois' two Regional Alzheimer's Disease Assistance Centers by the State Department of Public Health.

Nursing in the Rush curriculum was reconstituted under Luther Christman, Ph.D., a nationally known nurse educator from Vanderbilt University, where he had been the first male dean of nursing in the U.S. Christman came to Rush in July of 1972 and two months later brought from Vanderbilt Sue Thomas, Ph.D., soon to be Sue Thomas Hegyvary. Thomas was to help him in reviving nurse education at Rush, where there hadn't been any since the diploma (non-degree) school was closed in 1968, after the degree program became virtually obligatory.

The Christman and Hegyvary doctorates were in sociology and anthropology, which says something about the state of nurse education at the time; nurses' doctorates were in fields loosely allied with nursing rather than with nursing itself. Or they were ''content-free'' degrees in education. Christman set to work immediately to offer doctorates in nursing as such. Eventually, Rush offered a doctor of nursing science degree, the first in the Chicago area.

The Rush University nursing program combined education and practice, as the Presbyterian-St. Luke's diploma nursing school had done. Like the diploma school's teachers, its faculty were expected to practice as well as teach nursing. The program in this respect also imitated Rush Medical College, where teachers were also expected to be practitioners. The nursing program began in September of 1973.

Meanwhile, Christman's goal was to upgrade nursing to full professional status. The first step was to institute ''primary nursing,'' what Christman would rather call use of a ''physician-nurse team'' which takes responsibility for a patient from the time of entering the hospital.

This approach was a long way from the assembly-line, task-oriented nursing that dominated the field between the two world wars. During this period, when hospitals came into vogue as the place to go when you were sick, nurses divided various functions. One handled this, another that, and patients received all the expert attention that a new car got at an assembly plant.

For the Rush patient in the 1970s, however, the nursing process was intended to resemble more closely a work of art. Nursing services were put one by one on the "primary nursing" basis. Nurses were increasingly made responsible as professionals for patient care. Quality assurance was placed in the hands of nurses themselves, as it was for doctors. Sue Thomas Hegyvary led a federally financed study which gave norms for a self-checking process intended to put nursing as near to full professional status as possible.

At the same time the use of nurse's aides declined drastically. This was all right with Christman, who cites the inherent lack of opportunity for advancement of the nurse's aide along with the wastefulness of using one. Superiors have to spend too much time giving instructions to nurse's aides. A degreed nurse is more cost effective, he says.

The Rush program has been institutionalized and widely publicized as the "Rush Model for Nursing," which health care professionals have come from far and wide to observe. A half-hour educational film depicting the Rush Model for Nursing has had wide distribution in health care institutions throughout the U.S. and overseas.

This Rush Model covers everything about nursing at Rush from the presence of an all-registered-nurse staff to the system of compensating nurses. Primary nursing, in the hospital and at patients' homes, is central to it. There is a process of decentralized decisionmaking about patients' needs and centralized allocation of nurse personnel based on a daily gathering of workload information.

Teaching and the practice of nursing are merged, as we have seen; nurse faculty, the best educated of the Rush nurses, are Rush's managers of service, teaching and research, as is the case with medical faculty. Like doctors, nurses function as members of a fully organized, self-governing group with its own officers, bylaws, etc. Quality is assessed regularly by a team of nurses, most of them doctoral candidates. And finally, each nurse is paid according to demonstrated competence; indeed, no two nurses are as a matter of course paid the same salary, and thus financial incentives are present for each to improve herself or himself continually.

Creating and inspiring this whole Rush program has been Luther Christman, who is something of a grand old man of nursing in the U.S., lionized and anthologized and otherwise praised and blamed for his outspokenness. He has blamed nurses for their own subprofessional plight even as he has promoted an educational and professional upgrading of nursing itself. A member of the Institute of Medicine of the National Academy of Sciences, he has been a recipient of many other honors in his long career.

To attract undergraduate students in nursing and medical technology, Rush University has had to look to schools which, unlike itself, offer nontechnical undergraduate training. To help in this recruitment process, James Campbell established a network of colleges and universities to serve as feeder schools. Now 40 or so students a year transfer to Rush from network colleges in six states. The college network program thus has enjoyed moderate success.

In November of 1971, Rush introduced a second network, of patient care institutions, to achieve a vertical integration of patient care among a group of independent institutions. At the hub of this six-county network would be Rush itself, ready to handle tertiary-care cases referred by the other hospitals. This vertical integration would thus respect the capacities of each institution, whether small community hospital or tertiary-care medical center.

In the early seventies, Rush considered expanding its corporately owned hospital base to the northwest suburbs. But site approval suffered local-government delays, projected costs doubled, and plans were abandoned. In 1975, however, another opportunity arose to expand in the Far North Side of Chicago, and Rush assumed control of what became its Sheridan Road Hospital.

Meanwhile, Rush was sending residents and students (medical, nursing and other) to network hospitals for part of their training. These hospitals as a result were in a position to recruit staff from Rush residents and students. In addition, Rush teacher-practitioners offered continuing education programs in these network hospitals.

According to Campbell's plan, Rush and its network institutions were to serve 1.5 million people. If other Northern Illinois academic health centers did the same, each forming its own network and assuming its "fair share" of health care for the poor, a half dozen such systems could handle the area's health problems.

The Rush network began with four hospitals—Christ Hospital and Medical Center, Oak Lawn; Community Memorial General Hospital (now La Grange Memorial Hospital), La Grange; Swedish Covenant Hospital, Chicago; West Suburban Hospital Medical Center, Oak Park—and a clinic. By the mid-eighties, there were 18 hospitals.

The clinic was Mile Square Health Center, Chicago, which was part of an unfolding story of James A. Campbell's application of his "single standard" to health care for the indigent. In the late 1950s, after Campbell had integrated nonpaying with paying patients in Presbyterian-St. Luke's Hospital, the hospital's outpatient clinic for nonpaying patients remained, a relic. Its name itself, the Central Free Dispensary, breathed Chicago medical history. But it also breathed the double standard. Patients sat on long wooden benches waiting their turn and were called up by their first names. The Dispensary typified poor people's experience in receiving medical care.

Campbell as chief of medicine got it moved from its old quarters in the Rawson Building, diagonally across the street from Cook County Hospital, to the first and second floors of the new Jelke Building. Its name went the way of traditions no longer considered serviceable and, in August of 1961, it became the Presbyterian-St. Luke's Health Center.

Campbell put Dr. Joyce Lashof in charge of preventive

medicine at the newly named health center. He had known her when she was a staff physician at nearby Union Health Service. Lashof was later Illinois state public health director, U.S. Health, Education and Welfare undersecretary and dean of the school of public health at the University of California at Berkeley. Partly because of Lashof's influence, the clinic was modernized and its poor people's atmosphere sharply curtailed.

Then Lashof, on loan to the Chicago Board of Health, and Dr. Mark Lepper, who chaired the University of Illinois' department of preventive medicine, headed a Board of Health survey of health care for poor people in the city. Lepper had earlier headed the Municipal Contagious Hospital, and he had been a senior attending physician at Presbyterian-St. Luke's since 1958. He was to work closely with Campbell throughout the sixties and seventies.

Lepper and Lashof found huge gaps in health care in poor neighborhoods and recommended a massive public effort including setting up 24 neighborhood health centers throughout the city. Presbyterian-St. Luke's promptly followed through —the first of only two institutions to do so. In 1966 it joined a neighborhood organization in applying for a federal grant to begin a health center. This was the Mile Square Health Center, named after the Mile Square Federation, whose territory was the black ghetto community north and west of the hospital, bounded by Ashland and Western avenues and Kinzie and Van Buren streets. The center, modeled on the recently reorganized Presbyterian-St. Luke's Health Center, opened in 1967, with Lashof its medical director.

Overall responsibility for the center was Lepper's. He had joined Presbyterian-St. Luke's full time in 1965 mainly because Campbell and he agreed on single-standard care for the poor and how to provide it. Interviewed by Campbell, newly appointed president, for the chairmanship of medicine, he was hired instead as executive vice president for academic affairs. He saw the future of medicine as one system in the voluntary sector, and so did Campbell.

The concept enjoyed far from universal acceptance. Some believed in care for the poor primarily "to learn and experiment," as Lepper put it. It was "go down and do your thing, salve your conscience," he said. The poor "didn't dare call you. They didn't dare have any followup. If you weren't there, the next time they saw somebody else." Lepper felt used by County Hospital, for instance. He would make his rounds there, and they would say people got good care, although a patient's temperatures might not be recorded.

Campbell also argued against the double standard for educational reasons, as we have seen. He felt students should deal with people who will talk back to them, rather than with those who are captive by their poverty, who must accept whatever care is given them. He also argued that paying patients would profit by being seen by the eagerly inquiring young man or woman. In effect, why deprive the student doctor of paying patients and vice versa?

The Mile Square Center's approach was revolutionary because, like the Presbyterian-St. Luke's clinic, it guaranteed poor people the same treatment as paying patients. By now, of course, even the poor were paying, through Medicaid. But at public institutions they were still getting separate and not always equal care. Mile Square center patients, on the other hand, were sent to Presbyterian-St. Luke's if their physicians thought it necessary. There was no shunting them off to County Hospital. It was a care system that provided private practice continuity to "public" patients.

Campbell, who had grave misgivings about public institutions, wouldn't have had it any other way. Thus the new neighborhood health center mimicked the Presbyterian-St. Luke's center, and Campbell's single standard philosophy was expanded beyond Presbyterian-St. Luke's boundaries.

He tried to extend the concept citywide. He devised a plan that would permit indigent patients to use private hospitals throughout the city at public expense. Hospitals would each have taken its "fair share" of indigent patients and would each have offered single-standard care. The plan won acceptance from private hospitals but lost out politically, because of feared loss of jobs at public institutions.

Years later, in 1976, Campbell closed the Presbyterian-St.

Luke's clinics as the institution's last vestige of the double standard. Some said he was abandoning the poor, but he arranged for most clinic-registered patients to be accepted by private practitioners at Rush who agreed to forego their regular fees in exchange for public-aid payments.

The patient care network of which Mile Square Health Center was a small part was not as successful as Campbell hoped. Rush received tertiary-care referrals from its hospitals but mostly on a doctor-to-doctor basis rather than hospital-to-hospital.

The network's educational and training component worked fine, however. More than 3,500 students and 1,500 residents completed its programs, many then taking positions in network hospitals. Professional relationships developed from these contacts have worked to patients' benefit.

At the end of Campbell's first decade as president, in November of 1974, he recalled the comment 10 years earlier by John Bent, former chairman and president of the institution, that it was time for the hospital board to leave administration to the operating officers. This was a "most serious" redefinition of responsibility for management that imposed "a new kind of obligation," said Campbell in 1974.

Much had happened in 10 years. The $84 million budget was 10 times that of 1964. The hospital staff of 647 was 50 percent higher. Hospital capacity was up slightly, to 850 beds. It was soon to top 1,000 beds. The department of medicine, for instance, had gone from 140 members in 1970 to 244 in 1972 —a two-year leap of over 60 percent directly related to the revival of Rush Medical College. Many department heads had been recruited from outside, and many more teachers of basic sciences. Total faculty numbered more than 1,000. The combination of full-time and voluntary staff kept medical education "hand in hand" with medical practice. Research kept the enterprise scholarly.

Rush-Presbyterian-St. Luke's Medical Center had its own schools, its own university, its own hospital. It was dependent on no other institution, either for patient care or academic training, though it was "at the heart of a vast cooperative enterprise."

Indeed, during those early years, the glow of the enterprise suffused everything, partly because of the ample financial support available. Campbell's dynamism was the key to it all. A true scholar-physician, he took risks to achieve his vision. ("He gambled and won," said a critic.) Others were caught up in the excitement.

Jewish and Catholic trustees were added (there already were a few Catholics), so that the board more adequately represented the patient group. The additions also widened support for the institution, which was already considerable. Doctors in other institutions got the feeling that Rush had the money to do anything it wanted.

The best was yet to come. In November of 1976, the trustees approved Campbell's proposal for a $154-million capital development program to assure "the future of success" at Rush. The centerpiece of this Phase III of facilities development was to be a nine-story patient care facility linked to the existing hospital complex. A new Cancer Treatment Center was also to be built, also linked to the existing complex.

Of the $154 million, over $112 million would be targeted for patient-care facilities and over $10 million for academic. An additional $21.6 million would be sought for Rush University endowment, and another almost $9.6 million to support programs, especially research. Rush management was to raise $79 million internally and otherwise, including some by borrowing. The rest, $75 million, would come from private philanthropy.

This $75 million was ten times the goal of 20 years earlier, when the two hospitals had merged. Chairman Edward McCormick Blair and the trustee committee on philanthropy headed by Harold Byron Smith, Jr., pretty much agreed the money was there. It just had to be sought in the right way. Architect of the campaign was Sheldon Garber, vice president for philanthropy and communication and secretary of the trustees.

Early soliciting preceded public announcement of the campaign, as is common with major fund raising efforts, since early momentum is crucial. Among early major gifts was $1 million pledged by Trustee Robert C. Borwell which endowed a professorship in neurology to go with directorship of the multiple sclerosis center.

Another was $2 million pledged by the Woman's Board towards the new Cancer Treatment Center. The center was to be named after the Woman's Board. Other gifts followed, including $4.5 million from the John L. and Helen Kellogg Foundation for a national center for nursing excellence. By November 14, 1978, former President Gerald Ford was able to announce at a kickoff dinner that the Kellogg gift had brought the campaign to $38 million or "past the 50-yard line."

Later, at a 1982 dinner celebrating completion of the campaign, Ford was invited back to announce even better news, that the campaign had gone $8 million over its $75 million goal. "In football terms," he told his audience, "that's an extra touchdown and two points on the conversion."

There were 18 gifts of $1 million or more each. These totaled over $40 million. The campaign went over the $75 million mark with a major gift by Life Trustee Kenneth Montgomery. Medical staff members gave $5 million.

Eight endowed chairs were established and funding was completed for two others, bringing the endowed-chair total to 30. One of them was the James A. Campbell, M.D., Distinguished Service Professorship of Rush University, established with $2 million pledged by friends. It was "probably the only element of the campaign of which Campbell was unaware," said Sheldon Garber, whose performance in the campaign received high praise from Blair and Smith.

Spending the money was almost harder than raising it, however. The new Atrium Building had trouble from the start. This was the 222-bed patient care and surgical wing. At $75.6 million it was the most expensive project ever approved by the Illinois Health Facilities Planning Board, which had to certify that it was needed. Rush's application for the certificate of need was attacked vigorously by critics and competitors but was finally approved with only minor changes.

A heavily publicized controversy developed during the Atrium Building's construction. Rush, on the advice of a city planning official, bought and closed a short city block on

Paulina Street as a way to cut costs considerably. Rush acted with city council approval, and only after gaining the endorsement of the Medical Center District Commission. Rush made the purchase on November 29, 1978, for $97,500.

On January 2, 1979, the contractor barricaded the work site, as is customary in such projects, closing Paulina. Two weeks later, a blizzard struck. Streets became impassable. In the general frustration, the Paulina Street closing became a focus for critics of Rush at two neighbor institutions, Cook County Hospital and the University of Illinois.

A storm of protest and publicity ensued for months. Mayoral candidate Jane Byrne, riding the crest of the snowstorm that did most to elect her, stood by the Paulina Street barricades and promised, "The walls will come down." Rush was taken to court (not by Byrne), where it proved it had acted without deceiving any of the apparently aggrieved parties. Mayor Byrne eventually provided her own endorsement of sorts three years later, when she joined dignitaries on May 25, 1982, to help dedicate the once-controversial Atrium Building. Hard feelings in other quarters lasted several years after the 1979 uproar.

The Campbell era was drawing to a close. In June of 1983, approaching 65, he announced he was retiring as president of Rush-Presbyterian-St. Luke's Medical Center. No one had done as much for the reborn institution. He was the second founder of what had begun as Rush Medical College almost 150 years earlier. In September he was re-elected trustee, appointed consulting physician and reappointed professor, and was chosen for an honorary degree.

To the trustees on this occasion he spoke of the "new generation" of civic leaders and trustees, many of them present, who 25 years earlier had "caught the vision" of serving Chicago through "bold and enterprising" leadership. Typically, he spoke of what others had done. He was, after all, the man you couldn't head off as he went to hold the door. He urged them to remember that numbers weren't everything but compassion was, that everything they did was to be measured by the test of compassion.

He ticked off issues for their attention.

Corporate responsibility was one. How well would health care institutions be run? Rush had not had an operating deficit in his memory. The institution had generated its own working capital, thanks in part to how it was organized and run.

Another issue was competition among health care institutions. "Our faith," Campbell reminded the trustees, "lies in the private practitioner as the backbone of the institution."

Rush's ANCHOR Health Maintenance Organization, started 12 years earlier, was an example of successful competition. ANCHOR's membership was nearing 100,000. Campbell said he had urged the state to adopt the HMO principle for its medical welfare program, which he feared might revert to the "old dual system" of public health care for the poor because of cutbacks. This return to the old system would involve "enormous" financial expense and even greater loss to society because "class divisions" would be revived and "humanistic gains" would erode. It was James Campbell riding his single-standard horse again.

In three months, however, James A. Campbell was dead of a heart attack, and the era ended not with a bang but a thud. At a memorial service at Fourth Presbyterian Church on December 7, 1983, his name was added to the Rush-Presbyterian-St. Luke's pantheon. During his presidency the institution had not only kept pace but had taken a leadership position. Of greatest importance was the reactivation of Rush Medical College and the founding of Rush University.

The institution was caring for 30,000 people a year on an inpatient basis. Its total number of beds, having risen well over 1,200, was almost half again as great as when Campbell had taken office. Surgery had risen from 13,500 operations a year to 17,500. The medical staff had doubled, the number of residents and fellows had tripled. The number of employees had tripled. Rush with its 7,500 employees had become one of Illinois' top 25 private employers. Its budget of $300 million was 15 times the 1964 budget. Its assets had sextupled to almost $400 million.

At the memorial service, Dr. Mark Lepper was one of those who gave tribute.

"Without reservation," said Lepper, "I feel that under no other leadership would the resources available when Jim Campbell entered the presidency have produced anything remotely approximating the current Medical Center."

Campbell's goals, said Lepper, revolved around patients, "whose needs included both compassionate and technically excellent care." Care had to be the same for all patients, rich or poor, black or white. All socioeconomic and racial groups were to be served in a "fair share" manner, representative of the "entire metro-Chicago population."

Or as Campbell had told the trustees a few months earlier, numbers weren't everything, and everything had to pass the test of compassion.

New Leadership, New Directions
Rush-Presbyterian-St. Luke's
After Campbell

James Campbell considered the loss of a leader "a temporary matter," said Rush Chairman Harold Byron Smith, Jr., when Donald R. Oder assumed Rush's interim presidency. The true leader "assembles echelons of managerial and professional skill" ready to take up where he left off.

Smith had both Campbell and Oder in mind. Oder took over as acting president when Campbell left office in September of 1983 and remained until the following July. He was senior vice president and treasurer and associate professor in the College of Health Sciences and chairman of the Illinois Hospital Association. A former Arthur Andersen partner, he had headed several Rush projects, including the 1969 corporate reorganization.

He was thus in part the architect of the presidency as Campbell had filled it, namely as a physician–chief executive officer. The pattern thus set, the board wanted another physician active and respected in his field for its CEO. Given this requirement, Oder was out of the running for the presidency even if he did want it. But in his nine months as acting president, he made the most of it.

184

During that time, for instance, Rush set up its first occupational health centers in leased downtown space and considerably expanded its Rush Home Health Services. But the project that most reflected Oder's talents was Chicago Technology Park, announced in June of 1984, a few weeks before Oder passed the baton to Campbell's successor.

Chicago Technology Park was a $13.1-million high-technology industrial park financed mainly by city and state funds as an "incubator" for small companies, a place where individuals or small groups of scientists would work to develop marketable high-tech products. It would include a three-story, $8-million laboratory building for use by scientists and businessmen.

The park itself was 56 acres almost immediately west of the Medical Center District where Rush and the University of Illinois Medical School were neighbors not always on the friendliest terms. It was in part a tribute to Oder's "great skill, judgment, patience and humor" (cited by Chairman Smith) that the project was to be operated jointly by Rush and the University of Illinois.

Thus passed into apparent oblivion the unseemly squabbles of the late seventies over Rush's certificate of need for a new pavilion and the much publicized closing of Paulina Street —not to mention the invasion by County Hospital patients and doctors of the Rush emergency room. Under Oder the sometimes tense relationships between Rush and its neighbor institutions improved considerably.

Especially did he defuse the University of Illinois situation, which had sputtered and smoked throughout the Campbell incumbency. Oder managed to bridge the gap, making apt use of his skills as a listener with what an observer called a "down home" quality "masking an incisive mind."

During his brief incumbency, Oder "presided over development of new initiatives . . . while establishing and broadening cooperative understanding" with other institutions, the city and the state, Smith said.

Neighborhood relations also benefited from Rush's willingness to stay and invest heavily in the West Side, when as a private institution it could have moved. Its investment over the years of several hundred million dollars sent a message of stability to the area and the city. For instance, Rush was important to redevelopment of the area south of the Eisenhower expressway and east of Rush to the Chicago River. Center Court Gardens, for instance, a group of apartments and town houses, was developed by trustee Charles H. Shaw on Campbell's urging. Shaw also provided for transfer to Rush, at Rush's discretion, of the general partnership corporation which he formed to develop the property.

Rush was also active in the University Village Association, the neighborhood organization to its east, with its focus on community development, and in the West Central Association and West Side Project, with their thrust toward economic goals. Much of Rush's community involvement began in the sixties with start-up of the Mile Square Health Center. Oder maintained a strong interest in this involvement, which continued in health fairs, health screenings and other programs of Rush's community relations department. More important was Rush's hiring of blacks and Hispanics over the years, helping people to start careers who otherwise would not have had the opportunity.

Oder presided over the June 1984, commencement at which Campbell was posthumously awarded an honorary degree. A few weeks later, in July, Dr. Leo M. Henikoff took over as president praised by Chairman Smith for his "impeccable professional credentials and demonstrated managerial talent." Henikoff had been chosen after an eight-month national search. The curtain had fallen on the Campbell era.

Henikoff, a pediatric cardiologist associated for many years with Rush-Presbyterian-St. Luke's, arrived from Temple University in Philadelphia, where he had been vice president and dean of the medical school for five years. He had earlier served as associate and then acting dean of Rush Medical College and, what was to prove a particularly useful experience, as Rush's vice president for interinstitutional affairs with special responsibility for its patient care network.

A University of Illinois medical school graduate, Henikoff had done his internship, residency and fellowship training at

Presbyterian-St. Luke's Hospital in the sixties, with time out for Public Health Service work, eventually as chief of the service's congenital heart disease program.

In April, 1984, when he'd been elected by the trustees, Henikoff called Rush "second to none" in patient care. In his inaugural address, he emphasized integration of academic and patient care functions. By November he noted the reduced need for the hospital setting and said the Rush System for Health was going to move beyond the hospital. Patient care was still the priority, but the patient care setting would change. A year later, he foresaw a "wide range of new programs involving new technologies."

The primacy of patient care was reinforced before and after Henikoff took office, by Rush's outlay for the latest in medical scientific equipment. Rush was the first Chicago-area institution to operate a CT (Computed Tomography) scanner, the first to use magnetic resonance imaging, and one of the first to use a lithotripter—a machine that crushes kidney stones without surgical intervention.

Such technology fits the patient profile at Rush, where about half the medical-surgical beds are filled by patients referred by other institutions for tertiary or advanced care. For diagnosis and treatment of these patients, Rush keeps at hand the most sophisticated equipment.

The Henikoff presidency coincided with fallout from cost-cutting in health. Government, insurers, employers and other major U.S. buyers of health care had been cutting back for several years. Hospital occupancy levels declined, ambulatory care hit an upswing, same-day surgery became more common. The health care industry felt the pinch. Some fat was being cut, but much of the lost hospital occupancy represented care people needed but could not get because they had exhausted their benefits.

Rush began to hurt a little, though less than most comparable institutions. Still, Henikoff became convinced that strategy had to be threshed out at the top levels. He and Chairman Smith assembled an ad hoc trustee committee which met a number of times in the winter and spring of 1984 and 1985.

From the meetings came a new strategic plan and the groundwork for another philanthropic campaign.

Rush also laid off 200 of its more than 7,500 employees; they were the first layoffs in memory. In a letter to employees on April 8, 1985, Henikoff cited reductions in state and federal reimbursement for the coming year of $14.6 million and "continuing pressures in the private sector." Budget adjustments for the "tough period ahead" were "imperative." Counseling and placement help were made available for laid off employees.

In the same message Henikoff said Rush was "perhaps in a stronger position to weather these difficult times than any comparable institution anywhere in the country." Some hospitals would not survive, but Rush was upgrading facilities and acquiring technology and equipment to ensure not only survival but national leadership. The institution was to be "stronger than ever."

Ambulatory care would receive greater emphasis, though the hospital would remain central. A more aggressive approach was to be used. Rush-quality care would become available throughout the area. The strategy was to "bring medicine to the neighborhoods, rather than people to the hospitals," as former chairman John Bent put it.

ANCHOR Health Maintenance Organization (HMO) would be expanded. So would industrial medicine clinics and downtown satellite offices. A preferred provider organization (PPO) and an Independent Practice Association (IPA) form of HMO would be added. The limping patient care network would be redeveloped. The research program would be expanded.

Some of this was already happening. The ANCHOR HMO, a deliverer of prepaid health care services, was one of the first of its kind in Illinois. It was begun in 1971, after the HMO concept was put on the negotiating table by Rush's unionized employees. ANCHOR's share of patient care revenue, which at Rush is 87 percent of all revenue, rose sharply in the eighties —from 7 percent in 1980 to almost 25 percent in 1986. ANCHOR membership rose in this period from 38,000 to 130,000.

By the mid-eighties, alternative systems were proliferating.

Rush Contract Care, a PPO or Preferred Provider Organization, was launched in 1986 with 16 hospitals and the services of 1,000 doctors. Rush also participated in other PPOs—Voluntary Hospitals of America, for instance—as a way to reach as many patients as possible. Access Health, a more recent Rush project, is an IPA-type HMO and as such provides prepaid services through private physicians using their own offices and reimbursed on a per capita basis.

Two other alternative systems were the Rush Occupational Health Network, which serves over 3,000 employers in six Chicago-area offices, and Rush Home Health Services. In addition, satellite offices were established in two downtown locations: One Financial Place and River City. A "professional building within a building" was planned for the Northwestern Station Atrium Center.

All this evidenced a tilt toward ambulatory care. Indeed, ambulatory care and surgeries rose by the mid-eighties, while patient days (spent in hospital) declined. A Rand Corporation study of six successful academic medical centers cited Rush's entrepreneurial spirit. Henikoff attributed Rush's success to diversified programming and "broadened" community presence. ANCHOR HMO and more recent efforts plus advanced facilities and treatments had kept Rush competitive.

Rush had even gone into an entrepreneurial program of providing skills and services to health care institutions in three areas—pharmacy, home health care and accounts receivables management. This is ArcVentures, a for-profit subsidiary of Rush with a staff of 85 and 1986 revenues of about $8.5 million. ArcVentures operates the Professional Building pharmacy and a mail-order prescription service, markets at-home therapies and equipment, and provides billing and collection services to hospitals and doctors' offices. Its profits return to Rush while it promotes the Rush name and quality.

In the midst of all this bustle of alternative services and even of entrepreneurship, however, the heart of Rush has remained its private-practitioner medical staff. Its pursuit of health care was there from the first and remained the foundation of what Rush has tried to do over the decades.

Rush has remained competitive, but things have changed nonetheless since the seventies, when the sharpest disagreements among administrators were about how, not whether to spend, as Wayne M. Lerner, vice president for administrative affairs, recalled. The creative spirit remained from those days but not the wherewithal. The institution would fund 300 to 500 internal program requests a year, said John E. Trufant, Ed.D., vice president for academic resources and dean of the Graduate College and College of Health Sciences of Rush University. "We'd fund those things and raise the room prices," he said. When the money ran short in the eighties, "it was a much more difficult time."

Instead, there was soul-searching as payments dropped. The institution had to examine itself more than ever before. No one thought Rush would abandon its academic mission, but the new era had "severe impact," said Trufant.

Still, the institution prospered. The Campaign for the Future of Success closed in 1982 with $83 million raised. Then in 1986 came a resurgence of giving—$17 million, the most since 1982. That same year, 1986, a new Benefactors' Wall was erected on which principal contributors' names were inscribed.

In organ and tissue transplantations—liver, heart, kidney, bone, cornea and bone marrow—Rush became a national leader. In liver transplantation especially, Rush pushed boldly, and in less than a year was one of six or so U.S. institutions doing the procedure more than occasionally—one a week by 1986. It was a matter of deciding to do it and then recruiting "one of the best teams in the United States," said Dr. Henry P. Russe, dean of Rush Medical College and vice president for medical affairs.

Rush developed so-called specialty centers which enhanced its abilities in the most advanced treatments, including the Rush Cancer Center, the Multiple Sclerosis Center and The Thomas Hazen Thorne Bone Marrow Transplant Center. Rush also developed notable strengths in heart disease, orthopedics, psychiatry and geriatrics.

Rush's achievements have been recognized. Commemorating the 100th anniversary of Presbyterian Hospital in April of 1983, the Union League Club of Chicago gave Rush its Distinguished Public Service award for providing "the highest quality medical service to all segments of the community." *Business Week* and *Family Circle* magazines cited Rush for its leadership. A book soon to be published on top U.S. hospitals will do the same. Patients have frequently praised the care and attention they received. Among them is the president of Hyatt Hotels, who said in a post-stay letter, "You run one hell of a hospital."

Meanwhile, the patient care network developed new patterns. As specialization became more available, community hospitals began to do what only major referral centers like Rush had been doing. Henikoff had been Campbell's liaison with the hospital network in the late seventies and had a sense of what these institutions needed and wanted. He and others among the Rush leadership decided that Rush should work closely with these hospitals as they specialized, to help them increase their expertise. Rush would in effect work selectively to decentralize tertiary care activity while strengthening its communication and referral patterns with these institutions. The approach was being used with some success as 1986 drew to a close.

Possibly even more important was the interest of some network hospitals in merging with Rush. Before 1986 merger discussions had never moved past preliminaries. On the eve of Rush's sesquicentennial, however, at least two network hospitals were in negotiation, with agreements apparently imminent. Rush-owned facilities were already the most extensive among Chicago-area academic medical centers, and it had more operating beds than any other private hospital in Illinois. With mergers, the margin would widen even further.

The success of patient care at Rush has perhaps overshadowed an even older Rush tradition, the education of health professionals. This story began with recognizing the importance of medical education for community health. It should end with an appreciation of health professional education in all its aspects.

The figures tell the story. When Rush Medical College was reactivated in 1971, it offered only the doctor of medicine degree. In 1987, Rush University offered 30 degrees at three levels—baccalaureate, master's and doctoral. Rush University's four colleges—medicine, nursing, health sciences, and graduate college—have granted over 3,600 degrees in this time. Enrollment has remained for some time at about 1,150. About 350 graduate each year.

They are a remarkable variety. President Henikoff was only half joking when he told the trustees: "I hesitate to say that each of our graduating classes could go out and completely staff a small hospital, but if you added in the residents completing training each year, you wouldn't be very wide of the mark."

Rush has 33 endowed professorships, 10 of which came out of the Campaign for the Future of Success. Research awards topped 1,100 in 1986, for a record. The leading categories were in cancer, heart disease, immunology and neurology.

Henikoff had frequently mentioned the continued maturation or full development of Rush University when, within a year of his taking office, the trustees took him at his word and arranged an academic convocation at which he would be installed as president of Rush University. Campbell had regretted that in the rush of things he had never been installed as university president. He had realized it was an opportunity lost to tell the academic world about this new institution. The trustees were not about to make the same mistake again.

The installation was held in May of 1985. A national panel of speakers gathered to discuss "The Role of the Academic Health Center in the 21st Century." Honorary degrees were conferred. A touch of pageantry was provided. And more than 1,000 friends, colleagues and delegates from colleges and universities around the country settled back to hear Henikoff's inaugural address. For him it was the time to spell out his views on Rush's academic mission:

"In the late 1800s and early 1900s," he said, "people arriving in the new towns and cities of the West would ask if there was a 'Rush physician in town,' for such was our reputation in a time of greatly disheveled medical education. The public demanded quality.''

He went on to draw parallels with today's Rush, with its ''exciting and innovative educational program in nursing and in the allied health professions. Our Ph.D. candidates in science,'' he said, ''are part of a new and rapidly expanding research program, already demonstrating national leadership in several areas. Much remains to be done. Nurture and growth of these research efforts are essential to the maturation of Rush as a major health university.''

He emphasized ''the traditional role of practitioner as teacher'' and said it ''cannot be lost if we are to educate nurses and physicians and other health professionals who are humanists as well as scientists, who care about, as well as care for, the patient. In this regard,'' he said, ''our institutional philosophy of education in a health care environment serves us well.''

He voiced his fear ''that much would be lost if such education were to be removed from the bedside to the classroom.'' Rush's ''unique institutional position and philosophy'' enable it to maintain this approach to health education. Rush will not ''give up control of the academic health teaching environment, (namely) the hospital, to an entity that does not share (its) mission and ethic. . .''

He cited a trend towards ''separation of academics and health care delivery, brought about by current economic pressures.'' He called it ''not an unlikely scenario'' that universities might divest themselves ''of hospitals and perhaps medical schools.'' Rush's ''heritage and future,'' on the other hand, ''lie in the uncompromising intertwining'' of health care education with medical delivery ''in the forefront of patient care.''

Rush's base is in the health care system, said Henikoff. ''Our priority is the patient. In this we differ from most of our sister institutions. We have a unique role and a unique opportunity in this new era. It is up to us to make that opportunity a reality.''

President Henikoff spoke as successor to Dr. Daniel Brainard, the founder of Rush Medical College, who in his inaugural address reminded his audience of the great stake they had in the success of this institution. "The health, the happiness, the life of your dearest friends, and your own, may and will some day depend on the skill of some member of the medical profession," Brainard said in 1843.

Henikoff quoted him in 1985. He also quoted another of Rush's great men, Dr. James B. Herrick, who in 1912 said a hospital should have the "stimulus of instructing young, active, wide-awake" students and praised "the spirit of research" which freshens and enlivens education. "And yet no matter what view we may take," said Herrick, almost as if to head off any excess of enthusiasm for education and research, "the central figure is, and should be, the patient."

At Rush-Presbyterian-St. Luke's Medical Center for over a century and a half, the patient came first.

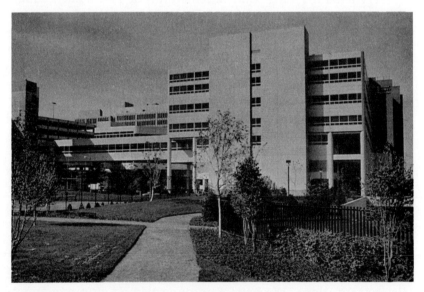

Rush-Presbyterian-St. Luke's Medical Center today.

Appendix I

AN ACT TO INCORPORATE THE RUSH MEDICAL COLLEGE

The Act of the Legislature of Illinois, Approved March 2, 1837, Entitled An Act to Incorporate the Rush Medical College

SECTION 1. Be it enacted by the People of the State of Illinois, represented in the General Assembly,

That Theophilus W. Smith, Thomas Ford, E.D. Taylor, Josiah C. Goodhue, Isaac T. Hinton, John T. Temple, Justin Butterfield, Edmund S. Kimberly, James H. Collins, Henry Moore, S. S. Whitman, John Wright, William B. Ogden, Ebenezer Peck, John H. Kinzie, John D. Caton and Grant Goodrich, be, and they are hereby created a body politic and corporate, to be styled and known by the name of the "Trustees of the Rush Medical College," and by that style and name to remain and have perpetual succession. The College shall be located in or near Chicago, in Cook County. The number of trustees shall not exceed seventeen, exclusive of the Governor and Lieutenant Governor of this State, the Speaker of the House of Representatives, and the President of the College, all of whom shall be ex-officio members of the board of trustees.

SECTION 2. The object of incorporation shall be to promote the general interests of medical education, and to qualify young men to engage usefully and honorably in the professions of medicine and surgery.

SECTION 3. The corporate powers hereby bestowed, shall be such only as are essential or useful in the attainment of said objects, and such as are usually conferred on similar bodies corporate, namely: In their corporate name to have perpetual succession; to make contracts; to sue and be sued; to plead and be impleaded; to grant and receive by its corporate name, and to do all other acts as natural persons may; to accept and acquire, purchase and sell property, real, personal or mixed; in all lawful ways to use, employ, manage, dispose of such property, and all money belonging to said corporation, in such manner as shall seem to the trustees best adapted to promote the objects aforesaid; to have a common seal, and to alter and change the same; to make such by-laws as are not inconsistent with the Constitution and laws of the United States, and this

195

State; and to confer on such persons as may be considered worthy, such academic or honorary degrees as are usually conferred by such institutions.

SECTION 4. The trustees of said College shall have authority, from time to time, to prescribe and regulate the course of studies to be pursued in said College; to fix the rate of tuition, lecture fees and other College expenses; to appoint instructors, professors and such other officers and agents as may be needed in managing the concerns of the institution; to define their powers, duties and employments, and to fix their compensation; to displace and remove either of the instructors, officers or agents, or all of them, whenever the said trustees shall deem it for the interest of the College to do so; to fill all vacancies among said instructors, professors, officers or agents; to erect all necessary and suitable buildings; to purchase books and philosophical and chemical apparatus and procure the necessary and suitable means of instruction in all the different departments of medicine and surgery; to make rules for the general management of the affairs of the College.

SECTION 5. The board of trustees shall have power to remove any trustee from office for dishonorable or criminal conduct; Provided, That no such removal shall take place without giving to such trustee notice of the charges preferred against him, and an opportunity to defend himself before the board, nor unless two-thirds of the whole number of trustees for the time being shall concur in such removal. The board of trustees shall have power whenever a vacancy shall occur by removal from office, death, resignation, or removal out of the State, to appoint some citizen of the State to fill such vacancy. The majority of the trustees for the time being, shall constitute a quorum to transact business.

SECTION 6. The trustees shall faithfully apply all funds by them collected, in erecting suitable buildings; in supporting the necessary instructors, professors, officers and agents; and procuring books, philosophical and chemical apparatus, and specimens in natural history, mineralogy, geology, and botany, and such other means as may be necessary or useful for teaching thoroughly the different branches of medicine and surgery; Provided, That in case any donation, devise, or bequest, shall be made for particular purposes, accordant with the object of the institution, and the trustees shall accept the same, every such donation, devise, or bequest, shall be applied in conformity with the express condition of the donor or devisor; Provided also, That lands donated or devised as aforesaid, shall be sold or disposed of as required by the last section of this act.

SECTION 7. The treasurer of said College always, and all other agents, when required by the trustees, before entering upon the duties of their office, shall give bonds respectively, for the security of the corporation, in such penal sum, and with such sureties as the board of trustees approve;

and all process against said corporation shall be by summons, and service of the same shall be by leaving an attested copy with the treasurer of the College, at least thirty days before the return day thereof.

SECTION 8. The lands, tenements, and hereditaments, to be had in perpetuity in virtue of this act, by said institution, shall not exceed six hundred and forty acres; Provided, however, That if donations, grants or devises of land, shall from time to time be made to said corporation, over and above six hundred and forty acres, which may be held in perpetuity as aforesaid, the same may be received and held by said corporation, for the period of six years from the date of any such donation, grant or devise; at the end of which time, if the said lands over and above the six hundred and forty acres, shall not have been sold, then, and in that case, the lands so donated, granted, or devised, shall revert to the said donor, grantor, or to their heirs.

Approved 2nd March, 1837.

Appendix II
Rush-Presbyterian-St. Luke's Medical Center

CHAIRMEN OF THE BOARD OF TRUSTEES

John P. Bent, 1956–1964*
George B. Young, 1962–1966*
Albert B. Dick III, 1966–1971
Edward F. Blettner, 1971–1974

Edward McCormick Blair,
1974–1978
Harold Byron Smith, Jr., 1978–

*Presbyterian-St. Luke's Hospital

PRESIDENTS

James A. Campbell, M.D.,
1964–1983
Donald R. Oder, Acting,
1983–1984

Leo M. Henikoff, M.D.,
1984–

RUSH UNIVERSITY DEANS

Rush Medical College

Daniel Brainard, M.D.,
1843–1866
James Van Zandt Blaney, M.D.,
1866–1871
Joseph Warren Freer, M.D.,
1871–1877
Jonathan Adams Allen, M.D.,
1877–1890
Edward Lorenzo Holmes, M.D.,
1890–1898
Henry Munson Lyman, M.D.,
1898–1900
Frank Billings, M.D., 1900–1924
Ernest Edward Irons, M.D.,
1924–1936

Emmett Blackburn Bay, M.D.,
1936–1940
Earle Otto Gray, M.D., Acting,
1940–1941
Mark H. Lepper, M.D.,
1970–1973
William F. Hejna, M.D.,
1973–1976
Leo M. Henikoff, M.D., Acting,
1977–1978
Robert S. Blacklow, M.D.,
1978–1980
Henry P. Russe, M.D.,
1981–

198

College of Nursing
Luther P. Christman, Ph.D.,
R.N., 1972–

College of Health Sciences
David I. Cheifetz, Ph.D.,
1976–1981
Bruce C. Campbell, Dr. P.H.,
Acting, 1981–1982; 1982–1983
John E. Trufant, Ed.D., Acting,
1983–1985; 1985–

The Graduate College
A. William Holmes, M.D.,
Acting, 1973–1974
David I. Cheifetz, Ph.D., Acting,
1974–1977
Mark H. Lepper, M.D., Acting,
1981–1982; 1982–1983
John E. Trufant, Ed.D., Acting,
1983–1985; 1985–

DEPARTMENTAL CHAIRPERSONS

Anatomy
Anthony J. Schmidt, Ph.D.,
1974–

Anesthesiology
Reuben C. Balagot, M.D.,
1967–1970
Max Sadove, M.D., 1970–1979
William Gottschalk, M.D., Acting,
1979–1980
Anthony Ivankovich, M.D.,
1980–

Biochemistry
Max Rafelson, Ph.D., 1960–1970
Howard Sky-Peck, Ph.D.,
1970–1978
Hermann Mattenheimer, M.D.,
Acting, 1978–1979
Klaus Kuettner, Ph.D.,
1980–

Cardiovascular Thoracic Surgery
Ormand C. Julian, M.D.,
1965–1971
Hassan Najafi, M.D., 1971–

Clinical Nutrition
Rebecca Dowling, Ph.D., Acting,
1986–

Communication Disorders and Sciences
Thomas Jensen, Ph.D., Acting,
1986–

Community Health Nursing
Iris Shannon, M.A., 1975–1976
Georgia B. Padonu, Dr. P.H.,
1977–

Dermatology
Frederick D. Malkinson, M.D.,
D.M.D., 1969–

Diagnostic Radiology and Nuclear Medicine
Richard E. Buenger, M.D.,
1968–

Family Practice
Philip C. Anderson, M.D.,
Acting, 1975
Erich E. Brueschke, M.D.,
1976–

General Surgery
Ormand C. Julian, M.D.,
1965–1970
Harry W. Southwick, M.D.,
1970–1985
Steven G. Economou, M.D.,
1985–

Geriatric/Gerontology Nursing
Lorry Gresham, R.N., 1977
Joan LeSage, Ph.D., R.N.,
1978–

Health Systems Management
Gail L. Warden, M.H.A.,
Acting, 1975
Richard A. Jelinek, Ph.D.,
Acting, 1976-1977
Bruce C. Campbell, M.B.A.,
Acting, 1978-1979
John G. Larson, Ph.D., 1982
Wayne Lerner, M.H.A., Acting,
1983-1984; 1985-

Immunology
Henry Gewurz, M.D.,
1973-1981

Immunology/Microbiology
Henry Gewurz, M.D.,
1981-

Internal Medicine
John S. Graettinger, M.D.,
1966-1970
Theodore B. Schwartz, M.D.,
1970-1982
Robert W. Carton, M.D.,
Acting, 1982-1985
Roger C. Bone, M.D.,
1985-

Medical Nursing
Sue Hegyvary, Ph.D., R.N.,
1974-1977
Ellen Elpern, M.S.N.,
1977-1979
Marilee Donovan, Ph.D., R.N.,
1980-

Medical Physics
Lawrence Lanzl, Ph.D., Acting,
1986-

Medical Technology
Marjorie Stumpe, M.A., Acting,
1986-

Neurological Sciences
Maynard M. Cohen, M.D.,
1963-1984

Harold L. Klawans, M.D.,
Acting, 1984-1985
Frank Morrell, M.D., Acting,
1986-

Neurological Surgery
Eric Oldberg, M.D., 1959-1971
Walter W. Whisler, M.D.,
1971-

Obstetrical and Gynecological Nursing
Ann Neeley, Ph.D., R.N.,
1974-1976
Claudia Anderson, Ph.D., R.N.,
1978-1981
Constance J. Adams, Dr. P.H.,
R.N., 1982-

Obstetrics and Gynecology
George D. Wilbanks, Jr., M.D.,
1969-

Occupational Therapy
Cynthia Hughes, M.Ed., Acting,
1986-

Operating Room and Surgical Nursing
Yvonne Munn, M.S., R.N.,
Acting, 1974
Joyce Stoops, M.S., R.N.,
1975-1976
Nellie Abbott, Ph.D., R.N.,
1977-1981
Joyce Keithley, D.N.Sc., Acting,
1982-1986; 1986-

Ophthalmology
William F. Hughes, M.D.,
1959-1975; Acting, 1976-1978
William E. Deutsch, M.D.,
Acting, 1979-1982; 1983-

Orthopedic Surgery
Robert D. Ray, M.D., Acting,
1969-1970

Claude D. Lambert, M.D.,
Acting, 1970–1971
Jorge O. Galante, M.D., 1972–

**Otolaryngology and
Bronchoesophagology**
Stanton A. Friedberg, M.D.,
1959–1973
David D. Caldarelli, M.D.,
1974–

Pathology
George M. Hass, M.D.,
1959–1974
Ronald S. Weinstein, M.D.,
1975–

Pediatric Nursing
Robert A. Lyons, M.S., Acting,
1975; 1976
Mary Beth Badura, M.S.N.,
1977
Jean Kaufman, Ph.D., R.N.,
1978–1979
Jean Sorrells-Jones, Ph.D.,
R.N., Acting, 1980–1981;
1982–

Pediatrics
Joseph R. Christian, M.D.,
1960–1985
Paul W. K. Wong, M.D.,
Acting, 1985–1986
Samuel P. Gotoff, M.D.,
1986–

Pharmacology
Paul E. Carson, M.D., Acting,
1974; 1975–1985
Henri Frischer, M.D., Ph.D.,
Acting, 1985–

**Physical Medicine and
Rehabilitation**
Jorge A. Galante, M.D., Acting,
1975–1980

Richard E. Harvey, M.D.,
1986–

Physiology
Joel A. Michael, Ph.D., Acting,
1974–1976
Robert S. Eisenberg, Ph.D.,
1976–

**Plastic and Reconstructive
Surgery**
John W. Curtin, M.D.,
1969–

Preventive Medicine
Joyce E. Lashof, M.D., Acting,
1970–1972
James A. Schoenberger, M.D.,
Acting, 1973; 1974–

Psychiatric Nursing
Jane Ulsafer, M.S., R.N.,
Acting, 1975–1977
Ann Marie Brooks, D.N.Sc.,
1978–1982
Karen Babich, Ph.D., R.N.,
1983–

Psychiatry
Paul E. Neilson, M.D., Acting,
1969–1971
Jan A. Fawcett, M.D., 1972–

Psychology and Social Sciences
David I. Cheifetz, Ph.D.,
Acting, 1970–1971; 1971–1975
David C. Garron, Ph.D.,
Acting, 1976
Rosalind D. Cartwright, Ph.D.,
1977–

Religion and Health
Bernard Pennington, B.D.,
Acting, 1975
Christian A. Hovde, Ph.D.,
D.D., 1976–

Therapeutic Radiology
Frank R. Hendrickson, M.D.,
Acting, 1970–1971; 1971–

Urology
Charles F. McKiel, M.D.,
Acting, 1969–1971; 1975–
Jack E. Mobley, M.D.,
1972–1973
Malachi J. Flanagan, M.D.,
Acting, 1974

MEDICAL STAFF PRESIDENTS

George W. Stuppy, M.D.,
1959–1960
Thomas J. Coogan, M.D.,
1960–1962
Richard B. Capps, M.D.,
1962–1964
Stanton A. Friedberg, M.D.,
1964–1966
Richard B. Capps, M.D.,
1966–1967
Rigby C. Roskelly, M.D.,
1967–1969
William S. Dye, M.D., 1969–1971
Frederic A. de Peyster, M.D.,
1971–1973

Philip N. Jones, M.D., 1973–1975
Maurice L. Bogdonoff, M.D.,
1975–1977
Milton Weinberg, Jr., M.D.,
1977–1979
Joseph J. Muenster, M.D.,
1979–1981
Robert J. Jensik, M.D.,
1981–1983
Andrew Thomson, M.D.,
1983–1985
Malachi J. Flanagan, M.D.,
1985–1987
James A. Schoenberger, M.D.,
president-elect

NURSING STAFF PRESIDENTS

Marcia Pencak, R.N., 1984–1985
Sandra McFolling, R.N.,
1985–1986
William Wiessner, R.N.,
1986–1987
Helen Shidler, R.N., president-
elect

PRINCIPAL OFFICERS

Harold Byron Smith, Jr.
Chairman
Roger E. Anderson
Marshall Field
Richard M. Morrow

Richard L. Thomas
Vice Chairmen
Leo M. Henikoff, M.D.
President

Bibliography

In writing this book, I have relied heavily on Rush-Presbyterian-St. Luke's Medical Center archivist William Kona, M.A. Without his help and that of his assistant, Mary Jane Kirchner, the enterprise would have been very difficult.

Among published authors I have depended most on Thomas Neville Bonner, whose *Medicine in Chicago, 1850–1950* gave me a valuable overview of the subject at hand.

Dr. Janet R. Kinney, biographer of Daniel Brainard and astute researcher, gave important help on the Brainard-Davis conflict and other aspects of those early years.

University of Illinois medical historian Patricia Spain Ward gave some good early advice; her article on Abraham Flexner was especially stimulating.

Dr. Frederic de Peyster supplied valuable audiocassette recordings and a history of the 13th General Hospital, among other items. Dr. Stanton Friedberg supplied a transcript of his conversation with Dr. Francis Straus and other materials.

Bruce Rattenbury, associate vice president for public relations at Rush, gave me reams of written materials and contributed greatly to my understanding of recent events. Some gaps in the 20th century history of St. Luke's Hospital may be explained by the unfortunate loss of some St. Luke's records at the time of its merger with Presbyterian Hospital. A bibliography follows.

BOOKS

Leslie B. Arey, *Northwestern University Medical School, 1859–1959: a Pioneer in Educational Reform,* Evanston and Chicago, Northwestern University, 1959, 495 pp.

Thomas Neville Bonner, *Medicine in Chicago, 1850–1950,* Madison, American History Research Center, 1957, 302 pp.

Norman Bridge, M.A., M.D., and John Edwin Rhodes, M.A., M.D., *Rush Medical College*, Chicago, Oxford Publishing Company, 1896, 154 pp.

James B. Herrick, M.A., M.D., *Memories of Eighty Years*, Chicago, University of Chicago Press, 1949, 270 pp.

Edwin F. Hirsch, M.D., Ph.D., *Christian Fenger, M.D., 1840–1902, The Impact of His Scientific Training and His Personality on Medicine in Chicago*, Chicago, 1972, 79 pp.

Hirsch, *Frank Billings*, Chicago, The Printing Department, University of Chicago, 1966, 144 pp.

James Nevins Hyde, M.A., M.D., *Early Medical Chicago, an Historical Sketch of the First Practitioners of Medicine etc.*, Chicago, Fergus Printing Co., 1879, 78 pp.

Ernest E. Irons, M.D., Ph.D., *The Story of Rush Medical College*, Chicago, 1953, Trustees of Rush Medical College, 82 pp.

Frederic Cople Jaher, *The Urban Establishment*, especially Chapter V, "Chicago," pp. 453-576, Urbana, University of Illinois Press, 1982, 777 pp.

Ruth Johnsen, R.N., B.S., M.A., *The History of the School of Nursing of Presbyterian Hospital, Chicago, Illinois, 1903–1956*, University of Chicago master's thesis, Chicago, Alumnae Association, School of Nursing, Presbyterian Hospital, 1959, 65 pp.

Rev. James DeWitt Clinton Locke, *Personal Reminiscences of the Diocese of Illinois, 1856–1892*, The Rev. R. B. Dibbert, editor, Chicago, Grace Church, 1976, 95 pp.

Marie G. Merrill, *The History of St. Luke's Hospital School of Nursing*, Chicago, 1946, 258 pp.

Bessie L. Pierce, *A History of Chicago*, Chicago, University of Chicago Press, 1937, 3 volumes: 1673–1848, 1848-71, 1871-93

The Pulse of Rush Medical College, the school yearbook, 1894 and 1895, Arthur Tenney Holbrook, Editor-in-Chief, 1894, pages not numbered; Samuel Omar Duncan, A.B., Editor-in-Chief, 1895, 376 pp.

The 13th General Hospital in World War II, 1942–1945, 62 pp.

ARTICLES, BROCHURES, ETC.

Emmet B. Bay, M.D., "Herrick as a Clinician," in "Joint Meeting in Memory of James B. Herrick" (of Institute of Medicine in Chicago and the Society of Medical History of Chicago, Oct. 14, 1954), *The Proceedings of the Institute of Medicine in Chicago*, 188–191

William K. Beatty, "Daniel Brainard—Pioneering Surgeon and Teacher," *Ibid.*, Vol. 34, 1981, 2 ff.

Beatty, "JVZ Blaney, Genial Chemist, Inventor and Editor," *Ibid.,* Vol. 39, 1986, 55–61, 111–118

Beatty, "Ludvig Hektoen—Scientist and Counselor," *Ibid.,* Vol. 35, 1982, 7–9

Beatty, "William Heath Byford: Physician and Advocate for Women," *Ibid.,* Vol. 39, 1986, 6 ff.

James A. Campbell, M.D., "Some Persons at Rush," *Transactions of the American Clinical and Climatological Assn,* Vol. 89, 1977, 162–171

Chicago Daily News, September 6, 1945, p. 2, "Chicago Doctors Hit the Beach First in Southern Japan"

Chicago Medical Society, *History of Medicine and Surgery and Physicians and Surgeons of Chicago,* Chicago, 1922

Chicago Tribune, June 13, 1950, "Doctors Dig Up Old Pranks at Rush '00 Party"

"Daniel Amasa Jones," Newton Bateman and Paul Selby, editors, *Historical Encyclopedia of Illinois,* Chicago, Munsell Publishing, 1906, pp. 926–928

Geza de Takats, M.D., "Parkinson's Law in Medicine," *New England Journal of Medicine,* Jan. 21, 1960, 126–128 (Presented Oct. 8, 1958, at annual meeting of the Mont Reid Society, Chicago)

John Milton Dodson, Sc.D., M.D., "The Affiliation of Rush Medical College with the University of Chicago—A Historical Sketch," *Bulletin of the Alumni Association of Rush Medical College,* 1917, January, May, September; 1918, January, August; 1919, April, November; 1920, February; 1921, February, June, October; 1922, May, August; 1923, January

Robert M. Hutchins, "The State of the University: a Report to the Alumni and Friends of the University of Chicago, Aug. 10, 1941," 20 pp.

C. Frederic Kittle, M.D., "Benjamin Rush—Heritage and Hope," *The Magazine,* Winter 1976-77, 46–51

Kittle, "The Development of Academic Surgery in Chicago," *Surgery,* Vol. 62, No. 1, 1–11

DeLaskie Miller, M.D., "Rush in the Past," *The Corpuscle,* Vol. 7, No. 8, May 1898, 271–274

Harold L. O'Donnell, *Newport and Vermillion Township, the First 100 Years, 1824–1924* (Vermillion County, Indiana), 1969

Walter L. Palmer, M.D., Ph.D., "Franklin Chambers McLean and the Founding of the University of Chicago School of Medicine," *Perspectives in Biology and Medicine,* Winter 1979, Part Two, S2-S32

Bruce Rattenbury, "A Generation at Rush—1964-1984," *The Magazine,* Fall, 1980, 8–22

Paul S. Rhoads, M.D., "James B. Herrick, M.D.," *Proceedings of the Institute of Medicine in Chicago,* Vol. 35, 1982, 3–6

Richard B. Richter, M.D., "A Short History of the Medical School at the University of Chicago," *Bulletin of the Alumni Association, School of Medicine, University of Chicago,* Vol. 22, No. 2, Spring, 1967, 4–7

Henry T. Ricketts, M.D., "Highlights in the History of the Institute of Medicine," reprinted in Nostalgia Corner, *Proceedings of the Institute of Medicine in Chicago,* Vol. 38, 1985, 84–86

John E. Rhodes, M.A., M.D., "The Making of a Modern Medical School: a Sketch of Rush Medical College," *The Medical News, Weekly Journal of Medical Science,* Vol. LXXIX, No. 20, Nov. 16, 1901, 761–767

"St. Luke's Hospital: 80th anniversary. 1865–1945," 1945

"St. Luke's Hospital, An Indispensable Institution," Chicago, 1923, Officers and Trustees of St. Luke's Hospital, 23 pp.

James P. Simonds, M.D., D.P.H., Ph.D., "Ludvig Hektoen: a Study in Changing Scientific Interests," *Proceedings of the Institute of Medicine in Chicago,* Vol. 14, 1942, 284–287

Samuel G. Taylor III, M.D., "Reminiscing about Medicine's Progress," *The Magazine,* Fall, 1977, 25–26, reprinted from *American Medical News*

The University of Chicago, the President's Report, July 1892 to July 1902, University of Chicago Press, 1903; succeeding editions, 1906–1924

Ilza Veith, "Medicine as an Academic Discipline at the University of Chicago," *Bulletin of the Alumni Association, School of Medicine, University of Chicago,* Vol. 32, No. 2, Spring, 1977, 13–18

Patricia Spain Ward, "The Other Abraham: Flexner in Illinois," *Caduceus* Vol. 2, No. 1, Spring, 1986, 1–66

George H. Weaver, M.D., *Beginnings of Medical Education in and Near Chicago, the Institutions and the Men,* reprinted from *Proceedings of the Institute of Medicine in Chicago,* Vol. V, 1925, Chicago, Press of the American Medical Association, 132 pp.

H. Gideon Wells, M.D., Ph.D., "Investigative Work at Rush Medical College," *Bulletin of the Alumni Association of Rush Medical College,* August 1922, 15–19

UNPUBLISHED MATERIALS

Arthur Andersen & Co., "Hospital Organization Study" of Presbyterian-St. Luke's Hospital, November, 1965, 26 pp.

Robert Cunningham, "The Making of a Medical Center," Chicago, 1980, 113 pp.

Frederic A. de Peyster, M.D., "The Great Medical Department of Lake Forest University, 1887–1898," Presidential address read before 71st annual meeting of the Chicago Surgical Society, May 21, 1971

R. Kennedy Gilchrist, M.D., *Its Been Fun: 1904–1984,* Memoirs, 294 pp.

Dora Goldstine, draft of projected history of St. Luke's School of Nursing, September, 1931, 82 pp.

Mark H. Lepper, M.D., transcript of interviews on April 24 and May 15, 1984, by Janis Long Harris

Rev. D. Clinton Locke, "History of St. Luke's Hospital to 1893," David Evans, editor, 1929, 30 pp.

Madeleine McConnell, R.N., B.S., *The Development of Nursing, St. Luke's Hospital, Chicago, a Memoir* (not dated)

Joan Willard Moore, "Stability & Instability in the Metropolitan Upper Class," a comparative study of the woman's boards of St. Luke's and Presbyterian hospitals, unpublished Ph.D. thesis, University of Chicago, 1959.

Presbyterian Hospital, Minutes of Board of Managers, June 15, 1938; June 9, 1939; September 7, 1939; February 26, 1941

Rush Medical College Alumni Association meeting, Atlantic City, June 18, 1963, audiocassette

Rush Medical College trustees' meeting (with meeting of medical staff, Presbyterian-St. Luke's Hospital), September 3, 1969, audiocassette

Francis H. Straus, M.D., "Some Medical Reminiscences," transcript of conversation with Dr. Stanton A. Friedberg, March 29 and April 1 and 2, 1980, 36 pp.

Andrew Thomson, M.D., "Remarks at Medical Staff Dinner," Nov. 1, 1984, 7 pp.

INTERVIEWS

Ralph A. Bard, Jr.
Evan M. Barton, M.D.
John P. Bent
Edward McCormick Blair, Sr.
John Brewer, M.D.
Mrs. James A. Campbell
Robert W. Carton, M.D.
Mrs. George Chappell
Luther P. Christman, R.N., Ph.D.
David W. Dangler
Frederic A. de Peyster, M.D.
Mrs. Herbert C. De Young
Albert B. Dick III
Stanton A. Friedberg, Jr., M.D.

Sheldon Garber
William F. Geittmann, M.D.
John S. Graettinger, M.D.
William Grove, M.D.
Sue Thomas Hegyvary, Ph.D., R.N.
William F. Hejna, M.D.
Leo M. Henikoff, M.D.
Ruth Johnsen, R.N.
Philip N. Jones, M.D.
Janet R. Kinney, M.D.
C. Frederick Kittle, M.D.
Joyce Lashof, M.D.
Mark H. Lepper, M.D.
Wayne M. Lerner, M.H.A.
Joseph J. Muenster, M.D.
Donald R. Oder, M.B.A.
Rhoda S. Pomerantz, M.D., M.P.H.
Henry P. Russe, M.D.
Barbara Schmidt, R.N.
Theodore B. Schwartz, M.D.
Charles Sheaff, M.D.
William D. Shorey, M.D.
Harold Byron Smith, Jr.
Irene R. Turner
John E. Trufant, Ed.D.
George B. Young, Ph.D., J.D.

Index